Vagus Nerve

Stimulate and Activate your Vagus Nerve by Effectively Reducing Inflammation, Anxiety, Migraine, Stress and other Chronic Diseases with Natural Exercises and Techniques and Unleash Your Body!

Eric Hermann

CW00732327

professional before attempting any techniques outlined in this book.

By reading this document, the reader agrees that under no circumstances is the author responsible for any losses, direct or indirect, which are incurred as a result of the use of information contained within this document, including, but not limited to, — errors, omissions, or inaccuracies.

Table of Contents

Introduction

Do you know what the vagus nerve is? For most people, the vagus nerve is something that isn't studied in schools, nor is it actually discussed in finer detail.

However, your vagus nerve provides stimulation to various organs within the body. Your vagus nerve is an integral part of your nervous system. It's more than just the longest nerve in the body, it's a nerve that helps control a multitude of functions.

But, how can you control your vagus nerve? That's what you're about to find out. In this book, we'll tackle some of the points of vagus nerve stimulation you need to know, and why it's so important.

I didn't know anything about the vagus nerve until recently, however I suffered from many different health conditions in life, several that oftentimes were almost too much for me to deal with. I started to do research into the vagus nerve, how it affects inflammation in the body, and why it matters. I discovered so many important elements I would like to tell you about them.

I was someone who thought the vagus nerve was just another nerve. Boy was I wrong! I learned what happens if your vagus nerve isn't properly stimulated, what happens if you have an inactive vagus nerve, and how you can pinpoint many conditions to a vagus nerve that isn't working.

I wrote this book to help you with understanding the different aspects of your vagus nerve, why it matters, and some important ways to help with vagus nerve stimulation, including how it will benefit you as a person, and how it can increase your health and wellness.

Chapter 1:
What is the Vagus Nerve?

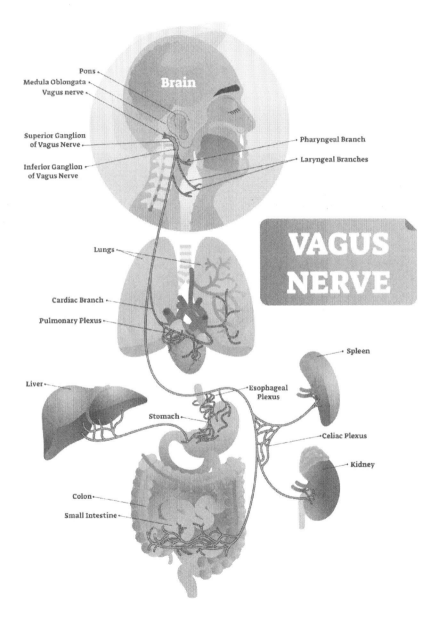

So, what is the vagus nerve?

Within our bodies, we have different nerves. There are nerves that extend from our brain called cranial nerves, and the vagus nerve is one of these 12 nerves.

However, it's more than just that. It's not only one of the 12 cranial nerves, but it's also the longest nerve of these 12. The name comes from the Latin word meaning wandering, since it tends to "wander" from our brainstem all through the organs in our chest cavity, our abdomen, and of course, our neck.

Now what's in this area? Our lungs, digestive tract, and heart are all parts of our chest and abdominal cavity. The vagus nerve has a big responsibility, and takes care of the vital functions of these different parts of the body.

It isn't just a giant nerve, it's a nerve with a whole lot of responsibility.

Long Nerve, Lots of Jobs

The vagus nerve is responsible of course, for your digestive, immune, respiratory, and cardiac systems. However, there's so much more than that. It's essentially a long nerve that helps the brain communicate with everything in the body, whether it be your heart rate, breathing, or other bodily functions.

There is a lot this nerve is responsible for, and for the most part, it takes care of the parasympathetic functions of the nervous system.

But what exactly does that entail? Read below to find out.

The Parasympathetic Functions

With the vagus nerve, the parasympathetic functions are controlled. There are two parts of our autonomic nervous system, the sympathetic, and the parasympathetic nervous system.

The sympathetic nervous system is responsible for all of the functions of our body when we're stimulated, and when we need to be on high alert.

Some of those functions include:

· Increasing your heartrate
· Gastrointestinal secretions
· Breathing increasing
· Pupils dilating
· More inflammation in the body
· Blood pressure increase

When we get hurt, our sympathetic nervous system kicks in. you get an ouchie, chances are you're scared, surprised, or whatever. Your sympathetic nervous system kicks in, and suddenly, you might notice your bruise get inflamed, or you might notice there's scabbing and puss forming. If you notice inflammation, that's a result of your sympathetic nervous system. Your blood pressure might increase as well.

However, your parasympathetic nervous system does the opposite of the sympathetic nervous system, which means, it's activated when the body is released. When your vagus nerve is functioning correctly, and you notice you're more relaxed, the following happens:

- Your blood pressure decreases
- Your heart rate lowers to its normal level
- Your breathing becomes less labored and deeper, more even
- The neurotransmitters that help get rid of inflammation get the signal to remove and reduce inflammation
- Your pupils relax
- Your body naturally secretes gastrointestinal juices to help with digestion
- Your body calms down and is not as tense

Usually, the parasympathetic nervous system kicks in when you're relaxed, or not on high alert, and when you're presented with a stressful situation, it goes on high alert.

But of course, that's not always the case.

It's More than Just Your Heart and Lungs

With the vagus nerve, it's much more than the heart and lungs. It's also, your sensory functions.

The vagus nerve is so long it can extend all the way around your ear canal, vocal cords, and underneath the tongue. Every time you stimulate this through these senses, it kicks in.

The vagus nerve handles the sensations you might feel in your ears, your throat, or even your mouth. When you sing, for example, it stimulates the vagus nerve, and it takes care of everything that's happening.

Your larynx, trachea, lungs, esophagus, and of course the heart are all controlled by this nerve too. Pretty much every function minus excreta is controlled by this, since the nerve itself extends all the way down to the colon.

But, if you have something near the root of your tongue, it also will stimulate the nerve here.

All of these sensations could be stimulated by your vagus nerve, so it has quite a bit of responsibility, and a lot to achieve.

Pretty much everything your body does can be attributed to your vagus nerve, so give your vagus nerve a pat on the back (or a proper stimulation) as thanks for all the hard work it puts in.

Now that we've discussed what it is, let's talk about some of the crazy things your vagus nerve can do.

What Can the Vagus Nerve Do?

The vagus nerve can do a lot, and if you're wondering just how far its influence extends, let's talk about it here.

- Your vagus nerve stems all the way from the brain, down to your colon, in a vertical fashion, and has at least some influence on the parts of the body there.
- Your vagus nerve sends communications directly from your gut to your brain, and it's part of the gut-brain connection, which we'll talk about later on.
- The vagus nerve is responsible for traveling down the body so the organs can do their jobs correctly.
- Have an upset stomach or just don't feel good? Your vagus nerve might be the culprit behind that.
- Your vagus nerve can be stimulated too much, or stimulated too little. When it's stimulated too little, it

causes vagal syncope, which is fainting, and that happens when your vagus nerve isn't properly stimulated.

· When vagal syncope happens, your vagus nerve basically overworks itself, will suddenly make your blood pressure and heartrate decrease by a lot, and suddenly, you'll fall down. This is sometimes caused by not stimulating it enough, or if you're under extreme levels of fear.

· There are ways for you to naturally stimulate this. While it is usually an involuntary response, if your vagus nerve isn't working right, it won't function correctly, which is why there are techniques to stimulate it.

Your vagus nerve is a huge nerve, one that goes all the way from the top of your body to the bottom, and you'll be amazed at how much your vagus nerve can do for you. In the next chapter, we'll discuss what your vagus nerve is responsible for in greater detail, and why it matters.

Chapter 2:
Why your Vagus Nerve is Important

So why is the vagus nerve important?

The better question is, when is the vagus nerve *not* important?
The answer is never. Your vagus nerve is so essential to your
well-being and happiness that you need to understand why it's
so important. We'll highlight the importance behind your
vagus nerve, and why making sure you have proper control over
it is essential.

Controls the Heart Rate and Blood Pressure

Let us discuss the first, and probably the most important reason
as to why our vagus nerve is important: our heart health.

The heart is a muscle, and each moment, there is oxygen-rich
blood pumped through your heart to various places in the body,
supplying the body with the nutrients it needs. If you don't
know the anatomy of the heart, the process is simple: the blood
goes to the heart to get oxygenated again and is sent out to
various parts of the body. Once that oxygen, and various
nutrients, are used, it's sent all the way back. This process
continues basically until you die or your heart stops working.

Pretty simple, right?

Your vagus nerve controls the rate of the heart, and your blood
pressure too.

Every time you breathe in, your blood pressure goes up, since you're taking in oxygen and that pressure changes in your blood. When you exhale, it lowers once again. Your vagus nerve is wrapped around the heart, and gives the heart electrical charges, just like a pacemaker.

Pretty cool, right?

Your vagus nerve is what properly controls how fast or how slow the blood is pumped through the body. If it's pumping too fast, it causes spikes in high, and then very lower blood pressure, the same with your heartrate.

If you've ever had an anxiety attack, you've felt the sudden heartrate, and then, the sudden drop. That's because, it can cause the heart to not pump enough blood through the body, resulting in fainting and loss of consciousness. In worst-case scenarios, it can permanently damage organs.

So yes, your heart is a major part of this. But we'll also talk about some of the other reasons why you shouldn't ever discount your vagus nerve, and what else it controls.

Breathing

It's debatable whether breathing, or heartrate is a bigger part of our lives. Personally, they're both incredibly impactful, but breathing is more than just taking in air.

Breathing is how you get the oxygen all over the place, and if an organ isn't getting enough oxygen, it dies.

Your organs can die if they're not given enough oxygen. When the body begins to shut down, a process called necrosis happens, and that's when oxygen isn't provided to your body, and the body part dies off.

Your vagus nerve is a part of this.

Your vagus nerve is responsible for making sure you're getting this vital air, so you can stay alive, and it encourages deep, even breathing.

If you breathe too fast, as a result of an anxiety attack, you're not providing enough oxygen to the body. Your oxygen levels decrease, the blood pressure and heartrate spike up, and then down, and that's what causes fainting.

Your vagus nerve controls this, and if you notice you're prone to either panic attacks, or fainting when you're anxious, it's best to understand that it stems from a vagus nerve suddenly being overly activated after not being activated up to this point.

Your vagus nerve also helps with relaxation. When you relax, your vagus nerve tells the rest of the body, "hey, it's time to chill" and the body follows suit.

So then, you'll breathe from your diaphragm. Diaphragmic breathing means you're breathing deep from your abdomen, rather than your shoulders, causing your belly to expand, and then go back to its normal size. This is in contrast to breathing from your chest and shoulders, which won't supply enough blood to the body.

So yes, your vagus nerve controls your breathing too, and it's a major part of making sure you don't breathe too shallowly, and to help supply the rest of your body with oxygen-rich air.

Controls Inflammation

What is inflammation?

It isn't just a redness of the skin or other areas of the body. It's an immune system response to various triggers in life. When you get a scrape or cut, suddenly you might notice it get red or swell. That's your immune system, and inflammation, working together to help treat the site of the problem.

However, not everyone's immune system works perfectly. This should only be triggered when there is some invader in the body, which in turn will release white blood cells in order to help fight this off. If there's just inflammation happening willy-nilly or a random stimulus, your vagus nerve steps in and controls this.

Your vagus nerve sends out neurotransmitters that help to reduce the inflammation in the body. These anti-inflammatory neurotransmitters control your immune system response. So, if you have any improper immune response, your vagus nerve should step in to help.

But, if your vagus nerve isn't stimulated, it can lead to inflammation when there is no reason to have inflammation. So basically, if that happens, you suffer from autoimmune conditions and inflammation that you can't control. For example, rheumatoid arthritis, celiac disease, and others can happen because there is too much inflammation going on in the body.

Your vagus nerve is responsible for this, and you should make sure it's working properly in order to stay healthy, and not stimulate the immune system when it doesn't need to be stimulated.

Gut-Brain Communication

Your gut, which is essentially all those parts of your body that help with digestion, all need to work together to properly digest your food in order to provide nutrients to the rest of your body.

Your vagus nerve provides direct communication from the gut microbiome to the brain of course.

Sometimes, if you're anxious or stressed, your vagus nerve will stimulate, which creates that "funny feeling" within the stomach.

But it's more than just that. Your vagus nerve controls the digestion of all kinds of foods, whether it be digestion in the stomach, or within the intestines in order to create excreta. If the vagus nerve isn't stimulated, it causes a lack of communication between these, which leads to gastritis, IBS, and ulcers occasionally too.

The vagus nerve also controls your allergies too. So, let's say you're allergic to peanuts. You eat a peanut, and suddenly, you start feeling sick. Your vagus nerve might stimulate the body once the allergic response is there and gets rid of the allergen.

It can tell the neurotransmitters causing inflammation that it's fine, you don't need it anymore, and the vagus nerve puts everything back in its rightful place. The vagus nerve might also control the gag reflex too, so if your body knows you're eating something you shouldn't, it'll communicate from the vagus nerve to the brain that you shouldn't be eating this, and it can cause reactions, whether it be throwing up or just not eating it at all.

If your vagus nerve isn't properly stimulated, it can lead to problems in your GI tract, so it's very important to make sure it's working as best as it can.

Relaxes the body

As we've said before, the vagus nerve controls your relaxation, where if you aren't in alert mode, it naturally relaxes the body.

The natural relaxation hormones are acetylcholine, which is a hormone that tells the body to chill out. The sympathetic nervous system, in contrast, secretes adrenaline and cortisol, which puts your body on alert, gives you more energy and affects muscle tension too.

When you experience high levels of stress, your brain will send out signals to different parts of the body. These different parts are controlled by the sympathetic nervous system, and with the vagus nerve, you also will have proteins and enzymes to be released which also relaxes the body.

It basically tells your body it's time to calm down and to not be on edge, which is good because if our sympathetic nervous system was always on high alert, we'd have lots of issues including blood pressure problems, heart disease, and breathing issues.

So, the vagus nerve works to help relax and restore the body, and promotes haling as well in times you need it.

Stimulates Peristalsis

Peristalsis is a fancy word that means the process of moving food through your digestive tract. Your esophagus, stomach muscles, and intestines all play a part in this process. When you swallow food, for example, the muscles used to push the food downwards, along with relaxing this, help get the food into your stomach. It prevents heartburn, indigestion, or food being lodged in your esophagus.

This slow pulsation is activated by the vagus nerve. It controls not only the pushing of this from the esophagus all the way down, but bile is produced by this, and your vagus nerve controls the bile that's secreted to help break down food.

If peristalsis doesn't occur, this may cause issues with bowel movements, food digestion, and even how your body handles secretions. Your stomach is controlled by this too, and if your vagus nerve isn't doing its job, that's a problem.

All of these different functions happen because of your vagus nerve. When your vagus nerve is properly stimulated, your body isn't in the "fight or flight" response, and instead, is relaxed, your breathing is easy, and you're happier too. When your vagus nerve isn't stimulated, it can affect everything from heart rate to respiration, to even how your body hands food. That's why, with proper digestion, everything is all squared away, and you can, with vagus nerve stimulation, create a better body, and promote wellness in all organ systems.

Chapter 3:
What happens to your Digestive Tract when you don't take care of the Vagus Nerve

Our vagus nerve is stimulated both voluntarily, and involuntarily. However, if it's not properly stimulated, many problems can arise. In this chapter, we'll go over how not taking care of your vagus nerve affects the rest of the body.

It can affect Your Hunger

Have you ever eaten a tiny amount of food and realized you're full? That's actually a sign of your vagus nerve in place. It controls all of the communication up and down the body, and the vagus nerve takes care of the hunger, along with the fullness signals.

When you have enough food, the signal for satiety goes all the way up to your brain, so it's basically telling your brain you're not hungry anymore after a meal.

There are also different neurotransmitters within our gut, like serotonin, along with ghrelin, and from there, these neurotransmitters send the feelings of fullness and hunger to the vagus nerve within the brain.

The perception of hunger, along with mood and stress levels, along with the activation of the inflammatory response in the body are all controlled by your vagus nerve. The signals that go from the brain towards the gut after you digest food and the digestive enzymes are all affected by your vagus nerve.

Your vagus nerve also works on pushing the food within your body out, which is a fancy way of saying it controls how much you excrete, and whether or not you're suffering from diarrhea and constipation or not.

This important pathway does control many different factors, including your health and weight, and here, we'll talk about as well what happens if you don't take care of your vagus nerve.

Obesity and Fullness signals

When you're obese, your vagus nerve isn't working as well, and the vagus nerve isn't as sensitive to the neurotransmitters for fullness. For example, you end up overeating and not getting enough exercise, which causes weight gin and obesity. However, there are even diets that can alter how your vagus nerve reacts to everything.

When you're obese it takes a lot more food to tell your brain that hey, you're full now. It also isn't a very strong fullness signal, so even if you do tell the brain you're full, the vagus nerve isn't working as strongly as it should. Oftentimes, if your vagus nerve is stimulated, it turns on these fullness signals, both in humans, and in animals. So, when you turn on the signal, you'll eat a whole lot less, feel fuller, and in turn, lose weight.

The Vagus Nerve and IBS Pain

It isn't just hunger and feeling full that can be controlled by this nerve. Irritable bowel syndrome, which is when you have pain from your bowel movements, can be altered and reduced with the help of your vagus nerve. If you stimulate your vagus nerve, it can help with pushing everything through your body, and reduce the pain that's there.

Vagal tone does control the motility of your body, and from there, you can use this to help with gastrointestinal pain, especially associated with dyspepsia, along with IBS.

The Vagus Nerve and Insulin Resistance

Insulin resistance is when you need more insulin to help break down the sugars in the body. For those with diabetes, or prediabetes, this can be a problem. This is mostly because, it takes much more insulin to reduce the blood sugar levels, and they tend to skyrocket.

Your vagus nerve has some control over your pancreas, which is where you secrete the insulin go help break down the glucose molecules in the body. When you're not eating correctly, it dulls the vagus nerve, which affects the performance of insulin in the body. It takes a lot more insulin to break this down, hence why for those with diabetes, it takes a shot in order to help reduce this.

There are also the factors of inflammation that play a part in this too, but insulin resistance especially happens when you're not taking care of the vagus nerve, and instead just eating whatever you want.

When you properly stimulate your vagus nerve, you'll be able to, with this as well, reduce your insulin levels in the body, and the blood glucose levels in the body too.

Gut-Brain Connection

Your gut and brain are directly connected by your vagus nerve. However, there is one chemical that plays a big part in stimulating your brain and gut together to help counteract hunger and to help move everything around.

This is called Lactobacillus reuteri, or also known as L. reuteri. This is a bacterium that's a part of your microbiome, which helps stimulate the breakdown of food as you ingest it.

The L. reuteri do this job by, when there is food here, your brain is then given the signal that hey, there's food here. From there, your gut health will be working, and in turn, it reduces the inflammation within the body.

This bacterium works to help the neurotransmitters come down, help to calm your gut and to make it so your body is properly digesting foods.

This also secretes oxytocin and dopamine in the body, which work to help the body through reducing the pain in the body, and also to stimulate blood flow. Dopamine especially is used in this way.

If the vagus nerve isn't properly stimulated, these neurotransmitters won't work, and from there, your body won't be able to fight off the inflammation that comes from your stomach acids, the foods that you eat, and the like. This causes "leaky gut," a condition where there's a permeability of the intestines where the bacteria and the toxins tend to "leak" through your walls of the intestine.

Leaky Gut and Your Vagus Nerve

Your vagus nerve is basically in control of making sure that any harmful substances are properly broken down through the function of neurotransmitters, and to also help with the peristalsis of the body.

Your digestive system helps to protect the body from harmful bacteria and substances. The walls of your intestines are essentially barriers that control the bloodstream and what's brought to the organs. The small gaps in your intestinal wall allow for these different nutrients to come into there, while also blocking the passage of substances that are harmful. The intestinal permeability is basically how easily these substances go through the intestinal wall.

When these junctions become loose, it essentially affects how permeable the gut becomes, which allows for toxins and bacteria to go into the bloodstream.

Your vagus nerve controls this inflammatory response, and helps with keeping everything tight. If the vagus nerve isn't properly stimulated, then, of course, this "leaky" gut happens, and from there, widespread and uncontrolled inflammation occurs within your body, and of course, causes autoimmune conditions to take root in the body.

For example, boating, sensitivities, digestive issues, skin problems, and fatigue all come about because of this.

If your vagus nerve is working correctly and is properly stimulated, it can help to reduce the inflammatory response, and in turn, reduce the inflammation in the body.

We'll go into further detail on inflammation in the next chapter, but understand that your gut isn't just a place where food is digested, it's also a location where a lot happens, and if things go wrong, it isn't fun for anyone.

Taking Care of the Vagus Nerve Through Foods

When you're looking to improve your vagus nerve, one of the first locations that we look at is of course, what you're putting into your body. When you have the "cafeteria diet" which involves lots of fats and carbs, it reduces the sensitivity of the vagus nerve.

However, by eating a lower-carb diet that's a bit higher in fat, such as keto but not as intense, it can help with that. There are ways to stimulate this as well through different tools and the like, but we'll talk about that later on because it's a little more complex than you'd think.

However, a lousy diet just makes you feel gross, and part of that is because your vagus nerve isn't being stimulated correctly. A good diet can help to counteract these problems, maybe even restoring it too. We'll highlight what you can do in later chapters to help properly stimulate the vagus nerve, but becoming mindful of what you eat, is very important, and it can help with reducing the instance of leaky gut, and also help with your microbiome.

Also, look at the bacteria in the body. Probiotics, whether through supplements or through the foods you eat, is incredibly important for vagus nerve health. The right foods you eat will help to change the body, and you'll realize that, with the proper stimulation and the right bacteria, you'll have a healthier body, and fewer instances of leaky gut, or gut issues.

Your gut and brain are connected, if only through this small nerve. Understand that what you do put in your body plays a major role in how you respond to the world around you, and how your vagal tone improves. We'll discuss more about vagal tone, and why it matters in Chapter five, but in the next chapter, let's talk about inflammation, and how your vagus nerve controls that, and how a lack of control affects it.

Chapter 4:
Inflammation, and what a Stimulated Vagus Nerve Can Do About it

Let's talk inflammation. Inflammation is something that happens within the body when there is a response to something that shouldn't be there.

Is all Inflammation Bad?

Not necessarily. In fact, inflammation is very important for making sure you respond to different stimuli within the body correctly.

With inflammation, you have either an injury, or a pain, or even an infection, and from this, you get more white blood cells, immune cells, and cytokines that are used for infection.

Inflammation is something that should be short-term, with redness, heat, swelling, and pain. But, in some cases, you might have inflammation happening within the body, without symptoms you normally don't notice.

When there is something in the body the brain recognizes as an invader, it starts the inflammation in the body. However, when not properly turned off, it can cause a lot of problems.

What conditions does it Cause?

Well, anything that yields an inflammatory response is a culprit here. For example, diabetes, heart disease, cancer, fatty liver disease, asthma, Chron's disease, IBS, and pretty much anything with inflammation as the cause is a part of this.

Food allergies and sensitivities are also seen here. Insulin resistance is another symptom of inflammation, hence why type 1 diabetes is often a result of inflammation in the body.

While some of the inflammation can be turned off quite easily, you'll realize that, with every single stimulus, it can actually make a lot of issues for people, and it can have a lot of problems that are very hard to fix if you're not careful.

People who are obese, or under a lot of stress, usually there is chronic inflammation there.

While you might notice it, most of the time you have to see a doctor to get some blood tests, including the C-reactive protein test, TMF alpha, and the IL-6, all of which are different chemicals appearing within the body whenever you have an inflammatory response.

So, What Causes It?

Well, there are many different causes here, and the vagus nerve is actually a part of this. When the vagus nerve is properly stimulated, it sends out the neurotransmitters to tell the inflammatory response that it's over, the invader is gone, you don't need to activate, which causes a reduced response.

But, with a vagus nerve that's improperly stimulated, it can cause you to have overstimulation of the inflammatory response within the body, resulting in insulin resistance, heart disease, obesity, and also other conditions.

This is partially caused by your diet of course. Eating high amounts of sugars, carbs, high fructose corn syrup, and consuming a diet that's riddled with junk food is a part of the reason why you might have inflammatory responses, and the solution, in that case, is, of course, a diet change.

If you're stressed, and continuously activating the parasympathetic nervous system, your vagus nerve will be affected too. This, in turn, causes an inflammatory response in the body too, and hence, diseases will come forth too.

But, it's more than just the sugars. It's also how your vagus nerve is stimulated. When your vagus nerve isn't working, it won't control the inflammatory response, and oftentimes won't control the signals to the brain. This will, in turn, lead to debilitating conditions in the body as we've discussed before.

In many instances, when we're continually reducing our "flight or fight" responses, the biological markers will help with reducing inflammation.

When you see a doctor for inflammation, chances are they won't prescribe medications for that. That's because the way to combat inflammation can't always be handled with medication, and oftentimes, medications cause more side effects than help to the body.

The vagus nerve affects your heart rate, and also acetylcholine, which is a tranquilizer that you can administer to yourself simply through inhaling and exhaling, and from there, your parasympathetic nervous system will be activated.

When you activate this, you're essentially encouraging the "rest and digest" or the "tend and befriend" actions in the body. The "tend and befriend" actions within your body, of course, are those neurotransmitters that are activated.

When you activate your vagus nerve, you're basically turning off all of those responses you don't need in the body, and it'll help with inflammation.

Arthritis and inflammation

One aspect of inflammation that your vagus nerve can help to combat, is arthritis. Arthritis is inflammation of the joints, resulting in pain when moving the body. There have been tests recently which connected your vagus nerve to the inflammation in the body.

Rheumatoid arthritis, in particular, is oftentimes curbed with enough stimulation. When you implant a vagus nerve device into your body, it reduces inflammation and improves the outcome because it helps to inhibit cytokine production.

Rheumatoid arthritis is a chronic disease that involves inflammation, and it affects many people each year, in fact over a million people suffer from this condition, and research has been done to help with combatting its effects.

Most immunologists and neuroscientists have used new technology in order to look for the exact neural information that will tell us where inflammation is caused. There is an "inflammatory reflex" that's been discovered our bodies have. This is actually a reflex causes cytokines to be produced.

Now cytokines are a part of increasing inflammation in the body, and are activated by an immune system response. Your vagus nerve essentially tells these cytokines to stop doing what they're doing, and it inhibits the overall production of these to help reduce inflammation in the body.

While more research needs to be done, it's been found that rheumatoid arthritis has been reduced by putting a tiny device in the body that triggers a chain reaction that helps to reduce cytokines, and thereby inflammation, creating a domino effect in the body when it comes to inflammation.

Most of the people can benefit from this right away are those with Parkinson's Alzheimer's, and Chrons, along with those with RA.

This device hopefully will help treat RA in the way it should, and reduce inflammation not just in animals, but also in people. It can help with improving your immunity.

While there is still more research to be done, especially on improving this, this is a great way to improve the lives of others. We'll discuss in more detail what vagus nerve stimulations via this device in a later chapter, but for now, understand that arthritic conditions, especially rheumatoid arthritis, are oftentimes curbed, and there is a lot this can do in order to reduce this condition in the body.

Bioletic integrative medicine is now taking on studies involving vagus nerve stimulation these days to help people understand and stimulate their vagus nerve in order to help them, and it will cause not only fewer side effects, but it also is cheaper than other options as well.

Improving Autoimmune Conditions

Autoimmune disorders are disorders that occur when your body is acting on automatic to stimulate the immune system. However, usually autoimmune conditions stick around because, while the threat is long gone, your body doesn't realize it. The parasympathetic nervous system isn't properly stimulated, and this results in fatigue, inflammatory conditions, and you feel terrible most of the time.

These are oftentimes considered conditions you can't see, but you can feel. For example, while you can't see someone all the time with lupus, this is an autoimmune condition, and it makes people feel fatigued and tired.

The autoimmune responses are inflammatory responses and they are used by the body to protect itself, but the problem is, protection oftentimes comes at a price.

But, your vagus nerve, when properly working, so work to help regulate this problem, making it easier for you to handle life. Autoimmune conditions don't need to lay waste to your body, but instead, by properly controlling all of this, you'll feel better, and much happier too.

So How do We Combat This?

Inflammation is something you can't always see. It's why many times, people with inflammatory conditions are those who have "invisible illnesses" since they aren't visible to the naked eye, and sometimes not even to tests either, but they're there, and they're wreaking havoc on the body.

The best way to work on improving inflammation in the body is to stimulate the vagus nerve. When properly stimulated, it can reduce the inflammatory responses in the body, helping you feel better, and reducing the instances of this. This is oftentimes much harder than you'd think because many of us live stressful lives where we're always in the "flight or fight" modes in the body.

But if you take care of your body, and work to combat inflammation, it can help with the body, and reduce the instance of overstimulation of the vagus nerve.

When the vagus nerve is properly stimulated, your inflammation seems to almost magically go away. It works in-depth the neurotransmitters within the body, in order to help everything properly work.

So yes, your vagal tone will affect the inflammation in the body, and in this section, we highlighted just what inflammation is, and why your vagus nerve is so connected with it.

Chapter 5:
Your Vagus Nerve and Mental Health

Did you know your vagus nerve plays a part in your mental health as well? It isn't just a physical sensation, but also a mental sensation. Sure, the fatigue and exhaustion are physical, but psychiatric conditions are affected by your vagus nerve, and in this chapter, we'll highlight just what they are, and how to properly understand the connection between your vagus nerve, and your mental health.

Your vagus nerve is a nerve that is connected to not only your brain and heart but to pretty much every upper body function.

The vagal tone you experience changes over time and vagal tone is a natural biological process within the vagus nerve. When your vagal tone is high and proper, it means you're relaxing from the stressful situation and calming down.

But your vagal tone plays a part in your emotions, and how your physical health happens. If your vagal tone is higher, then your physical and mental health will be higher too.

Your vagal tone and vagal response naturally reduce stress. Stress can make you experience both positive and negative emotions. A little bit of stress is healthy, but you should always respond to it after the stressful situation by calming down, but that's not always the case. Your vagal tone changes the brain's responses, stimulates the digestion of the body, and in general helps you to relax.

Relaxing is good for the body because if you're always stressed, you'll have trouble doing many things. Too much stress isn't good for you.

When We're too Stressed

Having too much stress isn't a good thing. Stress makes you depressed, anxious, and also angry, and it can affect your ability to make rational decisions, whether it's in daily life, or in the long run.

It also affects your dopamine and serotonin levels, both of which are neurotransmitters that handle our mood. Your vagus nerve handles the variability of this whenever it can, and when you're relaxed, you have more dopamine, serotonin, and you'll feel better.

For many of us, stress is a healthy way to accomplish things, but with the way life can be, it can be almost too much in many cases, and vagal tone is affected when we're stressed.

When you feel stressed, depressed, or anxious, your vagal tone changes, and oftentimes, you're more focused on negative emotions, and psychiatric conditions. Epilepsy also increases when your vagus nerve isn't properly stimulated.

You can measure this in different ways by looking at the EmWave2 waves which measure your heartrate variability, which shows your vagal tone too.

Higher vagal tone means everything is working better, and it can also help to stimulate your vagus nerve. You'll notice that when your vagus nerve is properly stimulated, you also respond to situations in a more positive manner, whether it be emotional, or physiological situations. Your brain and emotions are properly connected, and it can help offset the issues that mental illness causes to happen to you.

Your vagus nerve is the connection between your digestive system, brain, and other conditions. It also controls inflammation. But, your vagus nerve also handles mental health conditions, and there are many that your vagus nerve is attributed to.

What Conditions does a low vagal tone cause?

Low vagal tone, or otherwise known as your vagus nerve isn't properly stimulated, causes many different conditions in the body, and some of them are significant. Besides anxiety disorders and depression, it also is found in other types of conditions.

Degenerative mental health conditions, such as Alzheimer's and dementia, were found to be connected to your vagal tone. That's because, the inflammatory response in the brain isn't curbed, which causes degeneration of the nerve cells, and thereby this condition.

Migraines and other problems in the head, including tinnitus, are also attributed to your vagus nerve. When it comes to tinnitus, it's because your vagus nerve is very close to where your ear is, and actually wraps partially around the inner parts of the ear.

But, it's more than just these conditions. Addictions, eating disorders, personality disorders, even autism spectrum conditions are oftentimes attributed to your vagus nerve. That's because the mental health effects that come about due to the physical problems this causes can play a major role in your body's' ability to handle this.

Drug and alcohol addiction oftentimes happen because of this. It's because when the vagal tone isn't fully activated, it causes the body to seek out other alternatives since it's not getting enough serotonin in the body. For addicts, the happy feeling they get when they shoot up or take drugs, helps with this and can make them feel good, but it doesn't fix the problem of the vagus nerve not being stimulated, and oftentimes, it makes the problem worse.

But it isn't just serious conditions. Poor memory, mood swings and even mood disorders, MS, OCD, and several mental diseases and mental conditions can oftentimes come about because of this. Chronic fatigue is another problem too, and we'll get to that in just a moment.

Chronic Fatigue and Your Vagus Nerve

Your vagus nerve controls how your body handles certain conditions. When it's overstimulated, your body is fighting with the sympathetic nervous system, which is always putting you on high alert. But, if you're always on high alert, it'll make you feel thirsty and fatigued all the time.

This isn't just temporary tiredness either, it's oftentimes a serious condition, where you feel fatigued no matter what you do, and no matter how hard you try, it doesn't go away. This can be attributed partially to digestive and nerve health, but it does tie in to the vagus nerve.

So yes, chronic fatigue is caused by your vagus nerve, and it can make things very hard on you. It's also due to the breathing you're doing, because many people who have trouble breathing oftentimes suffer from improper vagal tone, and that's because people don't realize how impactful this can be on the body.

Brain Injuries

Having vagal tone that isn't properly stimulated does affect your brain and how it works. When your vagus nerve isn't properly stimulated, allowing you to get that air you so desperately need, your body won't get enough oxygen. Oftentimes, this causes vagal syncope, which is fainting involuntarily.

If you're not careful, you'll faint in a location that isn't ideal, which then causes head and brain injury. Sometimes, this trauma can be so bad you can't do anything about it, and instead, you're unable to perform functions in life.

This is probably the worst it can get, but it can negatively affect the rest of your body, even your life if you're not careful.

This is usually a more serious situation, but it's still worth mentioning, because many don't take into consideration what might happen if your vagus nerve isn't stimulated properly, and the truth is, a lot can happen if it's not, so remember that.

Vagal tone and Mental Health

Your vagal tone is part of your mental health, and a healthy vagal tone means better mental health. You can reduce inflammation, negative feelings, loneliness, even your instances of heart attacks or stroke if you're not careful.

Many people who have a higher vagal tone as part of a feedback loop between these emotions are oftentimes happier and in better physical health.

Healthy vagal tone also affects your social conditions too. You want to talk to other ore, and don't feel held back by depression and sadness when you have healthier vagal tone. You'll notice that you're much better off if you take care of your vagal tone, and you'll notice your vagal tone will improve your social interactions.

Humans are social creatures. We need to speak to others for the most part, or else loneliness sets in. we try to fill that void as much as we can, and even introverts need someone to talk to every now and then. Your vagal tone improves when discussing subjects with others, or just simply speaking in order to generate emotions.

When you're in a good mood, and your vagal tone is healthy, you'll notice that you have better human communications, and your bonds with others become more close-knit. That's because, you're taking care of your vagal tone, and are working to improve your vagus nerve stimulation.

Your vagus nerve does tell you about the "gut feelings" and the anxiety and fear you feel within the brain, and stress and depression are regulated via the vagus nerve, and your immune system plays a part as well.

When there are more cytokines in the body, you'll have better immunity, a happier body, and you're less at risk for developing mental health conditions. Cytokines also help with some types of depression, especially those with low mood, low motivation, and low energy. If you have more control over this, you'll feel better too.

What Can We do About This?

While you can't just "turn off" mental health conditions, stimulating your vagus nerve will help with this. By properly breathing, and taking the steps to calm the body down, it can help curb anxiety disorders, and stress-related to anxiety. It will help improve your mood.

Even just working with socialization can help with stimulation your vagus nerve. Communication has been proven to help with your vagus nerve, a properly stimulating it via communication will aid you in bettering your vagus nerve.

We'll give you the full rundown of what stimulating your vagus nerve will do for you and how to do it in later chapters, but this is how you do it, and understanding what you can do will help you immensely.

Chapter 6:
Your Vagal Tone, What That Means and How it Affects the Body

We've talked a little bit about vagal tone up to this point. But what is it exactly? Why does it matter? Read on to find out about vagal tone, and why it matters.

What is Vagal Tone?

Vagal tone is the scientific name for the vagus nerve responses to stimulation. It's how your vagus nerve is working, and how your heart rate, vasodilation, and constriction of the blood vessels, glandular activity, and respiratory rate are, and it showcases whether or not your vagus nerve is working to ensure that you're properly stimulated or not.

Vagal tone measures pretty much every parasympathetic action that occurs. So, if your vagal tone isn't working, you can definitely feel the effects, and it means you have a lower vagal tone.

For the most part, it's a measurement and a general idea of what's going on in the body, and for all of us, we all have a vagal tone that's constant, and we all have the same vagal output if everything's working perfectly and we're not pinned against one factor or another.

We were all, at the very beginning, blessed with the same vagal one. Theoretically, if we all are properly stimulated, we all could have the same vagal tone.

But there are a few reasons why people don't have a high vagal tone.

It could be because they don't have the proper stimulation of their vagus nerve. It could also be because their parents didn't have the proper vagal tone when they gave birth. Mothers do pass on their vagal tone to their kids, and this contagion of low vagal tone can be seen all throughout people.

We live in a high-stress, high-octane world. It's natural for most of us to have a lowered vagal tone when that happens. But you should work to have the highest vagal tone possible and work to properly stimulate yourself.

Your vagal tone is connected to many different parts of your body, and many different procedures, so it's only natural to have a high vagal tone in order to feel good and happy.

But, how is it measured? What happens when your vagal tone is low? Read below to find out.

Measuring your Vagal Tone

To measure your vagal tone, you can do this in a few different ways. Some people choose to go through vagus nerve stimulation, which is where you manually stimulate your vagus nerve through a device implanted in the body. We'll talk a little more about that later. But you can measure it through your vitals too.

For the most part, measuring it through your heart rate and respiration is the favored way. That's due to the fact the other procedures are much more invasive, and this will tell you right off what your vagal tone is, and why it matters.

The reason why your heartrate is used is because vagal tone and heart rate are intimately connected.

How so though? Well, your heart has a natural pacemaker implanted in the body, and that's through your vagus nerve. If your heart is healthy, this is naturally generating different impulses to move the blood through the body, and that's happening at all times.

When you sit in one place, your heart is beating. When you're running around, your heart is beating, and for the most part, the average beats per minute for a person is somewhere between 60-100. Sometimes, if your heart is very healthy, it requires fewer beats, so it beats much slower. If, however, you're not in good shape, it might beat more to get the blood going. When you're working out, you need the blood to pump faster, hence why the heart will beat faster if you're moving around.

However, it also is naturally turned off as well. When the heart rate is too high, your autonomic nervous system will then decrease your BPM, and if the heartrate is too low, as in the case of physical activity, it'll start to beat faster. This is done through electrical stimulation in your heart.

Along with that though, your autonomic nervous system is controlling the heartrate too.

This is all done without you realizing it for the most part.

The heart is controlled in two areas, whether it's the natural electrical pacing the autonomic nervous system has, or the autonomic nervous system working harder than the electrical activity that's going on right by the heart. Basically, these two things are working together so your heart beats correctly.

That's why your vagal tone is most accurately measured by your heartrate. If your heartrate quickly changes as a result of physical activity, and it doesn't suddenly make you feel too lightheaded to move, then your vagal tone is fine.

What about breathing though? How is that measured? Well, the next section will discuss that.

What About Breathing

Respiration is the other common way to tell you how good your vagal tone is.

That's because, breathing is when you take in the oxygen-rich air to supply to your heart, and then breathe out to get rid of the carbon dioxide produced.

But your heartrate changes when you breathe. Did you know that? When you breathe in, the heartrate increases, and when you breathe out, your heartrate will decrease. All of us have this happen, and this also happens in animals too. If you looked at your cat's heartrate, it would do the same thing it's doing in our bodies.

Your vagal tone for the most part should signify this, but sometimes, the vagal tone decreases. Our heartrate doesn't go up that much when we take in air, nor does it lower that much when we exhale. If your heart health is good, you'll have a great vagal tone, and this will happen all the time.

Those who are physically fit experience this as well. Because athletes are trained to control their heart rate, they are also in charge of their vagal tone. They can increase and decrease this at will depending on what their bodies have.

If your heart health isn't optimal, however your vagal tone will lower because of this, and that's a sign something's amiss.

Vagal tone is mostly related to your heart and respiration, but you could determine it through your diet too. But, that's more of a generalized inference, simply because, if you're just using digestive health to determine how healthy your body is, for the most part, it won't give you an in-depth look at the vagal tone.

Why does Vagal Tone Matter?

Well, knowing what your vagal tone says about you can tell you a lot about the state of your body. For example, if your heartrate is higher and your body is able to control it better, the better your vagal tone is. If you have a healthy heart with no complications, you can infer that your vagal tone will be the same way.

The vagal tone responds to different triggers too that you might not even know about. For example, if you feel depressed and sad, or maybe you have inflammation going on in your body, those with a higher vagal tone will have their bodies tell them about the triggers and the responses, and from there, you'll know when an anxiety attack, or a depression episode even, might come about.

In general, you can look for almost any abnormal sign that's happening in the body, and you could connect it straight to your vagal tone.

So, it does tell us more about what our body does than what we thought it could.

The vagal tone has a lot of control over our bodies, whether we like to admit it or not. Some of us experience both low, and higher levels of vagal tone when the situation calls for it.

Our emotions do also affect our vagal tone. If we're angry, anxious, or very stressed, our vagal tone decrease, and it affects the overall heartrate and respiration of the body. If you're feeling good, your vagal tone will be much higher. If you notice your body is doing well, then you'll feel much happier too.

Vagal Tone in Expecting Parents

This can even affect how parents respond to different stimuli too.

First-time parents especially feel the effects of this. With all the stress, anxiety, depression, and even lack of sleep they get, their vagal tone will be affected. That's why we see postpartum depression in women sometimes, and anxiety disorders can develop even after the baby's been born. There is also the fact that, if you're dealing with too much stress, it can affect your heart health and breathing rates.

Remember when they said stress would naturally kill you? It can. Stress affects your vagal tone. If you're not positive, optimistic, or combatting the stress effectively, your vagal tone suffers. This can affect your heart health and respiration. Hence why, those who are stressed tend to have a compromised immune system, tend to have heart conditions, and tend to have breathing issues. It's also why those who are stressed suffer from a variety of mental health conditions as well.

If your vagal tone changes for the better, you'll notice everything gets better. If you take the time to change your vagal tone, you'll notice you have better heart health, you'll have fewer panic attacks, less stress, and in general, a lot more happiness.

So yes, if you're an expecting parent, it can affect how you deal with the stress of having a kid. Some parents never recover, and some children are born with a lower vagal tone because of this, which can affect their physical, and mental health.

Serotonin, dopamine, and Your Vagal Tone

All of these are interconnected. Serotonin and dopamine are very good neurotransmitters for regulating emotions. If you're unhappy with life, depressed, stressed, and in general anxious or angry, your vagal tone lowers, and you won't have as much serotonin and dopamine in the body. However, if your vagal tone is better, you'll feel happier, or optimistic, cheerful, and you'll handle stressful situations in a much more positive manner.

That's because your neurotransmitters are all working with you instead of against you. So yes, your vagal tone will change how effective your neurotransmitters work, and it's why vagal tone is a direct indicator of the different levels your neurotransmitters are at, and why they matter.

Your vagal tone controls more than your heart, and it's imperative to remember this. If you're not looking at it like that, then you'll start to realize you're not as in control of your body as you should be, and those issues will develop.

Why Does This All Matter Though?

Think about it. It has a direct correlation between your own happiness, and how in control you are of your body. Your vagus nerve has a major job, and it's part of the reason why some people develop different conditions after a while.

For example, for those with recent bouts of depression, stress, and anxiety, along with other neurological and physical conditions, this shows up later on and can wreck your body.

Your vagal tone affects everything from respiration to your heart health and is responsible for quelling inflammatory response and keeping your immune system in check. If you are in control of your vagal tone, you'll have less of these issues develop in the body.

But, when you're not in control of your body and vagal tone, that's where immunity issues develop, where autoimmune conditions come forward, and where your heart health and respiration are thus adversely affected.

It also might be a temporary decrease as well. Those of us with acute depression and anxiety might notice the inflammatory diseases come up suddenly, rear their ugly heads, and then vanish like magic. That's normal.

However, those with treatment-resisting conditions might also struggle because their vagal tone is low. Treatment-resistant depression, for example, won't respond to different antidepressants and certain stimuli the same way, and oftentimes people don't even know why it happens. But, by stimulating the vagus nerve and working to better your vagal tone, you'll feel better, and it could help treat and help with controlling depression as well.

Can it Affect Compassion Too?

Some people say so. The parasympathetic nervous system does play a part in how your body handles different stimuli. The vagus nerve also does drive social connections, such as the motivations and behaviors we have when trusting others in affectionate, and cooperative manners.

Vagal activity does play a part in social connections and interpersonal behavior, but mostly in the realms of empathy, compassion, and of course, sympathy.

How though? Well, look at it this way. You can measure vagal activity through an electrocardiogram since of course, that's a way to measure a person's heart rate. When the heart rate is fully resting and kept low because of the vagus nerve, it will cause the heart to slow down. Your pacemaker is always going, but your vagus nerve puts the brakes on it. It's the main controller of our heart health.

Again, without it our hearts would beat so fast, we'd die. No joke.

The vagus nerve does this, where when we exhale it slows down, and beats faster to inhale, for the obvious reason of we're getting the blood to different parts when we inhale.

The strength of someone's overall vagal activity is measured by the difference in the heart rate when you breathe in, and when you breathe out. It is called respiratory sinus arrhythmia.

But, during these daily experiences of compassion, this will change. For example, let's say you're a kid, doing puzzles with another kid, and then playing with your parents. Children who do this will notice that, when you're more sensitive to others, it helps improve your focus. This, in turn, affects one's sympathy. It's been seen that vagal tone in kids who are older than three years that is higher will have more sympathy later on down the road.

Vagal tone from parents to kids does affect the concentration too. If a parent's working with a higher vagal tone child, they'll start to naturally meet in the middle, both of you understanding the other person.

But, if a parent is more authoritative, it means children will oftentimes not understand and have more compassion for others.

Those who were brought up in a more positive manner, where they were oftentimes understood and sympathized with, were oftentimes experiencing a higher vagal tone and compassion for others. That's because, vagal tone is a natural emotional regulator, and if you have a higher vagal tone, you're more sympathetic to other's suffering.

Vagal tone and mental health could play a part in this too. Those with lower vagal tone tend to experience depression and anxiety more and struggle with understanding others because of their own issues. Oftentimes they don't have a good emotional regulator in place as well, and their attention isn't fully focused on the subject or issue at hand.

When you feel compassion, your vagal tone goes up. It does make the heartrate go higher, and then go lower, and it does improve it, even slightly.

But, while this is still being studied, this does bring up a lot of points: how far does the vagus nerve extend? How much is out there that's controlled by this nerve?

The answer isn't fully known yet, and it may not be something we totally know for sure. But, understand that your vagal tone plays a part in this, from upbringing kids to even understanding others, and it's important to grasp that.

If you're reading this and wondering what to do next, well you can always go out and get your vagal tone measured. Or, you can stick around here, and if you already know your vagus nerve struggles, then start to learn about the different things you can do to help properly stimulate the vagus nerve.

Chapter 7:
The Exact Diseases a Vagus Nerve not Properly Stimulated Causes

The vagus nerve causes more and more problems than you'd think. In this chapter, we'll highlight the exact disease an improperly stimulated vagus nerve causes.

Esophagus Issues

For those with issues in their esophagus, whether it be cancer or otherwise, your vagus nerve may play a part in this. Your vagus nerve does have some control over your esophagus, which helps push food down the body. It's essentially how your food slowly moves downwards without choking you or going down too fast.

The vagus nerve does supply your esophagus with nerves, but for the most part, it also works with acid reflux. If your vagus nerve isn't properly stimulated, it can cause acid reflux, trouble swallowing, trouble eating foods, and it could even throw the food back up if you're not careful. Oftentimes, those who have issues with their vagus nerve can't eat large amounts of food very fast because it causes acid reflux in the body, or you end up regurgitating it later on.

You might notice nausea and vomiting more often too if you have a vagus nerve which isn't properly stimulated.

Gastroparesis

This ties into the esophageal conditions, and usually, the first sign of an improperly stimulated vagus nerve, or a vagus nerve that isn't working period, is gastroparesis. This is a condition where the stomach doesn't empty itself the way it should. That means food isn't going through the body in ways it should.

Usually, the following happens when you suffer from gastroparesis:

- Nausea
- Vomiting
- Heartburn
- Fullness feeling for no reason
- Acid reflux
- Bloating and IBS

The vagus nerve is responsible for peristalsis, which is the movement of the food within your intestines and other digestive organs. But, when you experience gastroparesis, there aren't any contractions to push the food along, which causes the food to sit there, making you feel sick, or even causing vomiting. Sometimes, you might even vomit up undigested food if this happens.

Most of the time, you'll feel too full to eat much food, and it causes weight loss, but also nutrient deficiencies too.

Those who suffer from gastroparesis also experience large amounts of abdominal pain and bloating too, which doesn't go away. Sometimes, it also leads to bowel movements which hurt, or a difficulty defecating.

Ulcers and Heartburn

This ties into gastroparesis as well, but because your neurotransmitter that is used to rest and digest your food isn't triggered, your food isn't properly broken down. This in turn, cause the stomach walls and lining to slowly degenerate, resulting in your blood sugar levels spiking, painful ulcers you might not even know are there, and a lot of acidity. It can break down the lining of the stomach and intestines too.

IBS

IBS, or irritable bowel syndrome, is a condition that makes bowel movements hard to do, simply because your stomach and other organs are so inflamed, or there's so much acid it makes the moment hard for the body.

Your body isn't properly digesting food, and this can feel awful. Everything from constipation, to even diarrhea, can happen due to this, and it makes eating certain foods a literal nightmare.

Sometimes this means significant amounts of weight gain or even weight loss, but you'll also feel tired, depressed, and very fatigued.

Cardiovascular Health

Certain cardiovascular conditions come about as a result of an improperly stimulated vagus nerve. Cardiovascular health and vagal tone are both intimately connected.

One of the main issues you'll have is bradycardia. This is what happens when your heart rate is slower than normal, where the body isn't telling the heart to speed up a little bit. This can make movements slower, and you feel fatigued in many cases.

The opposite of this is tachycardia, which is when you have a rapid heart rate. This is much more common than the latter, where your heartbeat is over 100 times a minute on resting.

The problem with that, is your heart isn't supposed to go that fast when resting, and if you're moving about, it can sometimes beat so fat you suffer from a heart attack. This will make you feel fatigued, overworked, and many times, it will cause the vital organs of the body to be affected too.

Anxiety disorders and panic attacks are also a part of tachycardia, and you might feel dizzy, shortness of breath, major chest pains, and heart palpitations. In severe cases, it causes unconsciousness, and sometimes, cardiac arrest for some people.

What's scary about this one, is that if you don't know whether you're at risk for heart conditions or not, you might not have any symptoms period. It might just happen, and that's because of improper vagal tone.

You could die if this is left unchecked, which is a scary thing.

This does make issues much more prominent, especially issues with physical activity. Most people with vagus nerve issues struggle with sanding for a longer period of time, and it makes movement harder. Other heart conditions can come about too.

Strokes do happen in some cases, but usually, this is oftentimes accompanied by other signs too, such as blood vessels that aren't properly dilated, and heart issues already known. Regardless though, part of the reason why you're having trouble is your vagus nerve, and that can negatively affect your lifespan in many situations.

Vasovagal Syncope

Another condition related to heart health is vagal syncope, and this is a condition where your body has a very rapid heartbeat, and then a very slow one. When you're sitting and suddenly getting up, you might feel faint, or it might happen when you're standing for long periods of time.

This happens as well when there's extreme heat, extreme stress, fear, sights of triggering things, and even just from dehydration of the body.

This is a heart condition, so it is commonly associated with the heart, since it does affect your heart rate and blood pressure, raising them heavily, and then suddenly dropping them. That sudden drop will make you faint.

It's a scary thing, and what they don't tell you about fainting, is that if it suddenly happens on an improper surface, it can cause head trauma, including fractures, skull damage, and concussions. So, there's is much more to this condition than just fainting willy-nilly.

Mental Illness

While mental illness isn't fully attributed to the vagus nerve, if you're not taking care of your mental health, your vagus nerve is affected, and vice-versa.

Even though the vagus nerve is a physical entity, our emotions are connected, and many times, if you're already feeling down due to what your body is doing to you physically, this will make you feel bad.

Think about it, if you're having digestive issues where you have no appetite, having heart conditions that don't make you feel good, and you're struggling with positivity and are feeling fatigued all the time because of your vagus nerve, it can cause depression and anxiety to spring up.

The vagus nerve helps to control our parasympathetic nervous system as well, which helps curb anxiety and eliminate the panic you feel when you have a panic attack. If it's not working at all, you'll notice you'll have trouble being happy, and it can cause anxiety to flare up as well. You'll also feel constantly tired, to the point where you don't want to do anything either.

While it isn't the direct reason, you're feeling that way, if you notice you're depressed, or feeling anxious a lot, chances are your vagal tone will show this too, and you can connect both of these together.

Inflammatory Conditions

The vagus nerve controls the inflammation, so if it's not working, or not activated at all, that causes inflammation to flare up, and it will cause inflammatory diseases. It isn't just arthritis either, but also ulcers especially peptic ulcers, sinusitis, asthma, Chron's disease, tuberculosis, periodontitis, ulcerative colitis, and other conditions that will happen over time. There are a number of inflammatory conditions that might come about, and autoimmune diseases such as celiac disease and allergies could be caused by a vagus nerve not working properly.

Inflammation is something that should go away after a while. Your vagus nerve is supposed to make sure that's the case, but when the inflammation is around for a longer period of time, that's when things become a problem. If you notice you have inflammatory conditions that aren't going away, then you should see someone for this.

Chronic Fatigue

This is partially caused by autoimmune conditions where you feel tired, fatigued, and don't want to do anything. We all naturally get tired when we work a lot, and have a bunch of things going on. But the problem is, if we always feel fatigued, that's when it becomes a problem. If your muscles always ache, or you're always sick or feel sick, or seem to always have colds or the flu, that's a sign that something is amiss. The problem is, most people don't even realize they're fatigued either.

For the most part, most of us just think it's mere tiredness, but that's not the case. A specialist will tell you right away it's more than just generalized fatigue that'll go away in a few days, but something bigger. If you constantly feel like you're tired despite getting enough sleep and eating properly, you should see a specialist. They can run lab tests and tell you what's going on.

They might not attribute it directly to the vagus nerve themselves, but if they tell you that there is something amiss, then it is your vagus nerve that's probably not being properly stimulated and that could be a condition.

Epilepsy

The vagus nerve, while not directly the cause of epilepsy, does control the instances of this, and a vagus nerve that's properly stimulated will reduce instances of epilepsy.

You can get vagus nerve stimulation to properly treat this. Seizures that are epileptic have been traced back to a vagus nerve that's not stimulated properly.

Epilepsy has many different symptoms, and Psychogenic nonepileptic seizures won't be benefitted by this. VNS is good for seizures that have a trace back to this.

While it isn't usually the main reason why seizures happen, it can help with controlling seizures as well.

There are other factors that might affect seizures, and there might be other methods used initially to treat them. For example, if you take medications frequently, or if you have other factors in your lifestyle that affect these seizures, you might get trigger management treatments first before we go to VNS.

However, there is a connection between the vagus nerve and epilepsy that's treatment-resistant conditions that might be in place. Epilepsy specialists will discuss this with you when you look for treatments, and if you've tried multitudes of drugs and other treatment, they might suggest the vagus nerve as the primary culprit.

However, there are other problems as well that might attribute to the vagus nerve along with epilepsy. If you suffer from breathing and heart issues with epilepsy already, then this could be attributed to vagus nerve conditions.

Sleep Apnea

Sleep apnea is the condition where you stop breathing for a small period of time when you sleep. Usually, this means you're snoring while sleeping, and you wake up tired and fatigued every single day. While sleep apnea has a variety of reasons behind it, from grinding your teeth to stress, your vagal tone could play a part in how your sleep patterns are and could attribute to sleep apnea in a few people. If your sleep apnea is getting worse, it may be due to the vagus nerve being unstimulated.

When the vagus nerve isn't properly stimulated, the pathways aren't open, and your nasal passages are oftentimes blocked. That means, for small periods of time, you're not breathing, and then, you suddenly start to snore or breathe heavily to make up for this. If your vagus nerve isn't properly working, then this can come about, but this tends to be a much rarer circumstance than other means.

However, if you've tried drugs and you don't have any clear indication for a reason why, it might be due to your vagus nerve not working correctly.

Chronic Breathing Issues

Breathing issues are another problem that could be due to your vagus nerve not functioning properly. Remember your vagus nerve is responsible for controlling breathing and the fibers that move through the respiratory tract. When your vagus nerve isn't stimulated enough, it might cause issues with breathing, and you might not get enough oxygenated air.

Sometimes, if it's not stimulated enough properly, you breathe from your chest, which means you're not supplying the heat with air. This can cause you to feel numb, faint, and oftentimes could put you into cardiac arrest too. Breathing plays a key part in your survival, and if you're not breathing correctly due to your vagus nerve, it can pose major issues.

The longer your vagus nerve isn't stimulated, the more extreme the problems become in the future. Not only that, conditions such as asthma and other breathing issues will come about because of this, so it's imperative that you take care of your vagus nerve, so you can breathe better and live longer.

Sensory Problems

Senses can be dulled due to your vagus nerve too. Hearing issues, taste issues, and even auditory conditions can come about due to your vagus nerve.

Your vagus nerve is responsible for the epiglottis and the palate, which is in charge of your ability to taste foods. If your vagus nerve isn't stimulated, some foods may not have a taste, and you might have trouble eating them. It might also cause you to develop bulimia too, or sensory issues with eating too. Sometimes, the acid reflux will make you taste acid flavoring when you eat food, which isn't fun either.

The ear is another part of your sensory organs that are affected by the vagus nerve. If it's not working, chronic ear pain, hearing problems, hearing loss, or even ruptured eardrums might occur too. You could develop tinnitus too, which is ringing in the ears, and that's not fun.

It doesn't affect the other senses as much, but these two are a big part of understanding what you're consuming, and two very important parts of the world around you. So, it shouldn't be discounted.

Don't Waste time, Take Care of your Vagus Nerve Today!

If this hasn't proven to you yet that your vagus nerve is a big part of your life and needs proper stimulation, then you should take the time and look at yourself in a physical sense. For example, if you know your body has strange medical conditions that don't have a cause to attribute to them, it's time to see someone to help you unlock your vagus nerve.

If you've already seen a myriad of doctors already, and not a single one of them can pinpoint a direct cause, then it's got to be your vagus nerve. There is probably not enough stimulation, and though you might not even realize the impact of this, it will affect your full potential.

But it isn't just making sure you live up to that potential. The diseases, conditions, and other problems that develop are affected by your vagus nerve, and in some cases, autoimmune conditions and heart trouble reduces greatly just from stimulating your vagus nerve.

If you've tried to do something about it and it hasn't disappeared, or it got worse over time, then it's time for you to see a specialist. There is vagus nerve stimulation, which is an invasive process that happens. However, if you want to take care of your vagus nerve on your own, that's possible too. I do recommend doing that first, and from there, if you know there are problems and they're not getting better, then call for a specialist.

But, not taking care of your vagus nerve leads to trouble, and this chapter showed just how bad it could be if you don't take care of it right away, and do something about it before it's too late.

Chapter 8:
Different Simple Actions You Can do Each Day to Stimulate your Vagus Nerve

So, what can you do to stimulate your vagus nerve in simple ways? There's a lot actually, and this chapter will help you dive in and learn some of the simple actions you can take each day to stimulate your vagus nerve. We'll go over what they are, why they matter, and how you can start with these today.

Cold Water and Cold Elements

The cold never bothered you anyway, right? Well, the cold is actually a wonderful way to stimulate your vagus nerve and improve your vagal tone.

Some of us don't like the cold, especially cold water, or cold showers. But, the vagus nerve does get stimulated when you're cold.

Do you ever notice you feel less sluggish and tired when it's cold? Sometimes, we feel down and tired during winter months due to the lack of sunlight we're exposed to, but oftentimes, we sleep better and sleep longer because of our vagus nerve.

When we are doing this, it does stimulate the parasympathetic nervous system. Sometimes, when it's unbearably hot, this kickstarts the body to burn more energy to help keep everything cold. Sometimes, this is why you experience more anxiety depression, and sleep issues.

It's because you're exposing yourself to too much heat, and not enough cold to change it up.

When the body's exposed to cold, there is a nerve cell in a place called the cholinergic neuron, and this is also strengthened through choline, found in eggs. This cell is important, because it transmits the chemical acetylcholine to different organs within the body, whether it be slowing the heart rate down, lowering your breathing rate by making you breathe in deeper, and in general, promotes physical relaxation.

This cell is good for keeping the parasympathetic nervous system activated, which means it contracts the muscles and then releases them, dilates the blood vessels, increases bodily functions, and of course, lowers your breathing and heart rate.

When the body's exposed to cold, it decreases the fight or flight response in the body, lowers your heart rate, and anxiety and of course, helps to improve the parasympathetic cavity in the body, making you feel better, and more relaxed as a result.

Sometimes, you can simply go outside when it's cold for about a minute and feel the refreshing effects of it. But, if you live in a climate that's incredibly hot currently, simply go into the shower and take a cold shower very quickly.

It doesn't have to be long. Sometimes, taking a hot shower, and then for 30 seconds before you leave, turn on the cold, it can help too. You can enjoy the relaxing hot shower, but then stimulate your vagus nerve with the cold water.

It won't be pleasant, but then again, would you rather suffer from the conditions of an unstimulated vagus nerve. This isn't the end-all solution, but it's a good way to give the vagus nerve the wakeup call it deserves.

Sometimes doing this in the morning is a good way to wake the body up, and get it ready for action.

Singing and Humming

Singing along with humming is wonderful ways to stimulate your vagus nerve. It's simple to do, and the idea behind it is simple to understand as well.

When you hum, your sound is coming from the vocal cords in the back. The vagus nerve wraps around the vocal cords there, and when you hum, it stimulates them, making you feel relaxed and happy.

Some people hum voluntarily, and sometimes people hum when they're doing things that make them happy, or they feel relaxed. Some even use humming during meditation too because it helps to naturally relax the body.

This is a big part of intent-focused meditation, and we'll discuss that in a later chapter. But, if you're not a fan of meditation, you can still attain the great benefits of humming just through your daily life.

What about singing though? Singing is an activity most people don't do because we feel self-conscious when we sing. But, if you sing, you naturally stimulate the vagus nerve which is right by the vocal cords. It also makes you feel good, and will naturally stimulate your body too.

Some people sing when they're scared, and when there's something bad going on, they'll do this. That's because it relaxes them and helps them feel less anxious during these stressful times.

The next time you sing, think about how you feel. Does it make you feel good? Then yes, it helps a lot.

There is also the factor of endorphins. Whenever you sing, the endorphins in the body naturally increase, improving your vascular system, because you have to take more air not you, and then expel more air out as well.

Some people notice how they feel when they sing, and it's a way to naturally calm them down. If you're not good at singing, sometimes you do this when you're driving, and it magically makes you feel better, allowing you to unwind. Singing releases serotonin and oxytocin, which make you feel happy, and reduces stress in your body. They're, of course, part of your parasympathetic nervous system, so it'll naturally help you relax, sleep, and feel blood.

Singing also increases vagal tone in the body, because your breathing varies over time, and you'll be able to regulate your emotions pretty easily too.

Singing allows for you to regulate all this, making you feel good and happy.

Laughing

Along with humming and singing, we of course have laughing. People encourage others to laugh because it'll make them feel good, but did you know it also stimulates your vagus nerve too?

Sometimes, when you laugh uncontrollably, you stimulate the entire body, including your vocal cords, which again stimulates your vagus nerve, and it also allows you to release many of those happy hormones too, including serotonin and endorphins.

Funny things that make you happy secrete both of these, so if you can find something you personally enjoy that makes you burst out in laughter, then enjoy it. Some people like to watch funny cartoons when they feel down, and while it might seem like a temporary high, it's a good thing to have if you're feeling down.

Physical Contact

Physical contact is healthy for the body, and good for your vagus nerve too. I understand some of us aren't keen to touch, but physical contact, especially hugging helps the body a lot.

Sometimes, after a long day, a hug will help release these chemicals, and it communicates to the brain that it's okay to relax here.

Have you ever had a day that was so stressful you felt like wanting to scream, and then second you got home, you relaxed because your pet was right there, waiting for you to come home? That makes us all feel great, and it's an example of feeling relaxed because of a stimulation. You'll instantly feel better, and much happier too. These chemicals, including serotonin and oxytocin, secrete when you engage in physical contact, and it makes you feel great.

If you don't live with a loved one or don't have someone you can hug every day, that's okay. Sometimes, hugging a pet, or even a stuffed animal when you're stressed out provides the same results, and it will change the way you feel as well.

Washing your Face

Washing your face helps with vagus nerve stimulation. But why is that?

When you wash your face, you're naturally engaging your diving reflex. This is a reflex both humans and animals have, and it's like what dolphins use when they got into water that's either deep, or has a colder temperature. It will start to constrict the vessels, and oftentimes slow down the heart and relax the body. By doing this, it pushes the oxygen towards the brain and the heart, and a blood shift happens where your organs are increased. The heartrate naturally slows, and your vagus nerve is stimulated.

This happens every time a marine mammal dives into the water, and for humans, by simply washing your face, you can achieve the same effects by exposing our faces to water.

While we can't dive directly into the water, unless we have a pool nearby or something, but we can wash our face to help with stimulating the vagus nerve. You can do this every morning. By washing your face for a small period of time, this will naturally activate the vagus nerve and also activate both the immune system and your digestive system.

Some people do this another way too.

The process is simple: what you do is you take some ice cubes, put them in a Ziploc bag, and from there, hold them to your face. It'll be cold, but as you do this, breathe in slowly. You might notice your heart rate slow down at this point, and your body naturally relaxes. I don't suggest holding it there for too long, but in those moments of panic, this could prove wonderful to try out.

Look at Your Diet

Your diet plays a big part in vagal tone. Remember what we said about leaky gut and digestive problems that come about because of an improperly stimulated vagus nerve? Well, one of the simplest ways to start with this is to make some dietary changes, and we'll highlight what they are below.

Have Probiotics

Probiotics are bacterial cultures that you take not the body either through a supplement, or through dairy products. Having these products will supply your gut with healthy bacteria to keep it alive and thriving.

Also, if you have a lot of bad bacteria in your diet, introducing probiotics into this will help with taking out some of the bad bacteria, and introducing the good bacterial cultures back into the fray. The one downside to this, is sometimes it can be a little bit too much for some people since they are potent, and a little bit goes a long way.

If you don't want to take a singular supplement, incorporate more cheese and probiotic-rich yogurt into this. That way, it helps push the good bacteria into your body, and eliminates any of the bad bacteria that might be there.

Natural Foods

Natural foods are the way to go. Diets that are organic, raw, wild-caught, or pasture-raised are good to have. You should read the labels as you go along to ensure you're eating proper foods.

Some people might choose to go keto in this case, which is the low-carb high-fat diet that is great for your body. This will help reduce the excess gluten and carbs in the body.

But you don't have to go full keto if you don't want to. A big part of the reason why you might have digestive issues and a vagus nerve that's not properly stimulated is due to the lack of consuming whole, natural foods. Some people eat foods with tons of dyes in them and lots of chemicals which cause leaky gut. But foods that are whole and natural will help.

Keto is recommended, but even just reducing your carbs, even a little will aid you in your bodily health, and also stimulating the vagus nerve too. Some people also do well with only a moderate level of protein, because eating too much turns he protein not glucose, which means you're supplying too much sugar to the body.

But, if nothing else, cut out the processed foods, the foods with chemicals in them, and also any foods that might have toxins you're unsure of having. This way, you can keep your vagus nerve properly stimulated and under control, so it's activated and helpful.

Remember your gut and your brain are intimately connected, so you should make sure you take the time to properly take care of your body so you can have a healthy vagus nerve.

Consider Omega-3s

Omega-3 fatty acids are a big part of your vagus nerve stimulation. Omega 3 fatty acids are an essential fat necessary for improving the body for a variety of reasons.

For starters, it's a required fat, but not something the body naturally produces. Omega-3 fatty acids help provide nerve health and supplement wellness there, which means it can help with improving your nervous system, including the vagus nerve itself.

You can get omega-3s from fish, or even from eggs and other types of fatty food. It's a healthy fat that promotes brain health, wellness, and generalized happiness.

Omega-3 is great for a vagus nerve in particular because it helps provide strength to the nerve cells, including the different parts of your vagus nerve. But, there's more to that. it helps with your mental health as well.

It can improve cognitive wellness, and improve functions in terms of thinking and brainpower too. If you have a leaky brain, anxiety, or even depression, this can help offset some of these problems. Brain fog is another common issue that can be resolved with omega-3 supplements.

Omega-3 fatty acids are also known to help increase your vagal tone, vagal activity, and also reduce the heartrate variability in the body, which leads to a properly stimulated vagus nerve. By having more fish in your diet, it'll help with vagal activity, along with the dominance of the parasympathetic system.

The easiest way to get omega-3 fatty acids is from supplements, and if you're someone who doesn't like to eat a lot of fish, this is a good way to do it. Usually, 1-2 supplements a day gives you your daily recommended amount, and it'll help with your body and your mind.

Fish oil, which contains a lot of omega-3 in it, has been known to help the body and your health of course. Adding this to your diet will help with improving this in the body, and adding this type of food to your body will benefit you too.

The Impotence of Fiber

While we did discuss fiber as a key part of vagal tone, most don't realize how important this can be. Many studies don't touch on this, but fiber is incredibly important for gut health, and it does a ton for the body.

For starters, fiber will improve your GLP-1 levels, which means that the hormones that communicate between your vagus nerve and your brain will be properly stimulated.

GLP-1 also helps with improving the rate in which the stomach empties out the food you consume. It's good for improving bowel movements along with offsetting different digestive problems too.

Fiber can be achieved either through your diet or through supplements in the body. It's recommended to have fiber as well because along with fat, it keeps you fuller for a lot longer.

If you want to get fiber through your diet, consider having a lot of greens. These are high in fiber for the most part minus starchy potatoes and other tubular vegetables. Otherwise, you can take a supplement that contains this.

Regardless though, fiber is a great way to improve vagus nerve stimulation, and it's something that should be considered.

Acupuncture

Acupuncture is a simple, yet effective way to stimulate your vagus nerve. The thing is, humans have been able to naturally do this for many years, and it's something that ancient Chinese medicine takes pride in. Acupuncture is great for the nervous system because of many of the benefits you get from this.

For example, since you can get acupuncture in different areas of the body, you can get it right where the vagus nerve is located. Your ear, for example, is one of the best places to get acupuncture treatment in order to stimulate this.

How does acupuncture stimulate your vagus nerve? Well, the little needles that are inserted into the body are right by the vagus nerve, which means it'll properly stimulate this nerve directly. If you go regularly, it will stimulate this.

Does acupuncture hurt though? Not necessarily. Some people might find it uncomfortable, but others might not even notice.

The needles in acupuncture are so small that you won't realize you even have them in there.

Acupuncture is great for reducing stress and tension as well, a common symptom of improper vagal tone, so if you go to an appointment every now and then, it can help with reducing this.

If you have vagus nerve issues, the practitioners can put needles in the areas that it feels are needed. For example, your feet, ears, neck, and also near the sides of your chest are common areas, and for your neck and ears, that's right near the vagus nerve, so when the needles are inserted it'll basically wake up the vagus nerve, and get it ready for action.

Acupuncture promotes full-body relaxation, along with immunity-boosting. It also improves deep breathing, something we'll discuss later on. But of course, breathing in a deep and controlled way combined with proper stimulation of the vagus nerve will help with vagal tone, and increase this as well.

This is one of the best and most natural ways to stimulate your vagus nerve, and if you want something that feels good, and is incredibly worth your while, I highly recommend going. Even just 30-minute sessions will change your vagal tone.

Intermittent Fasting

Intermittent fasting is a way to stimulate the vagus nerve. This is one of the diets that not only stimulates this naturally but also works to promote better brain health and wellness.

Most people don't think fasting every now and then would change the vagal tone of the body, but it really does. Why is that though?

First, let's talk about intermittent fasting. This is fasting which entails you only eating during some periods of time during the day. For example, you might not eat for 16 hours, but then you'll eat for 8 hours. You might choose to eat between 10 am and 6 pm, and during that time, you consume your daily caloric intake. You don't eat during the fasting periods.

Some people might even do full-on fasts periodically throughout the week, such as every other day fast, and then after that, eat shortly afterward. This is a bit harder however, since it requires discipline, and ensuring you eat enough food the day before the fasting period.

You might wonder how not eating stimulates your vagus nerve. Let's look at the basics. Eating involves consuming calories. Fasting involves doing the opposite of this.

When you don't consume your calories, your heart rate goes up, since it has to work harder to accommodate for the lack of food in the body. Your metabolism in turn will plummet, and these are the actions that stimulate the vagus nerve.

Your vagus nerve stimulates when the metabolism goes down, and it will help relax the body a little bit. When you're not metabolizing as much food, the body tends to be more relaxes.

Over time, it will progressively relax the body, and also help with stress reduction as well.

It isn't just good for stimulating g the vagus nerve however, you can utilize intermittent fasting to reset your metabolism as well.

What's the best schedule for this though? That's ultimately up to you. Ideally, people get results from 12 hours of feeding, and then 12 hours of wasting. However, you have to monitor yourself and make sure you don't eat everything at once.

If you eat all your calories in one shot, within a short period, you'll feel sick. Eating progressively a little by little, every few hours at that allows for you to enjoy your food.

Some people consider skipping meals since this is a simpler way to do it. However, I suggest listening to the body on that one. If you haven't eaten enough, you'll start to feel famished, and that's not fun.

The problem with intermittent fasting is most people start off doing more than they should be. For example, they'll try an all-day fast instead of just skipping a meal or setting up an eating schedule. The problem is, this can be too much, to begin with. The other problem is people won't eat enough food. During the feeding period, you need to eat your caloric limit. But even more so, you should be working to ensure you eat enough high-protein foods and also some high-fat foods too, since this will keep you fuller for longer.

You need to eat the proper amount of calories, and also make sure you're not just consuming processed garbage. Try to eat organic foods instead if you can.

You should take it slow, start out with maybe skipping one meal and going from there.

The beauty of intermittent fasting is that you can set up the means to do this. However, you should understand that if you just suddenly stop intermittent fasting, it causes issues with digestion, and it can make you feel sick.

Not only that, if you're using intermittent fasting in order to lose weight, this does cause the you-you effect where you'll gain all of that weight back, which king of stinks if you're trying to lose weight.

The best way to do intermittent fasting is nice and slow. Don't try to do it all right away, but instead, take it easy, don't be stressed about this, and do it in a way where you're able to handle all of this, and take on whatever it is you want to do with vagus nerve stimulation.

Gargle it Out!

Finally, another simple exercise we can do is gargling. Why would gargling help with stimulating this? It might seem odd, but gargling does wonders for your vagal tone, and it has the same effects as humming or even singing in some cases. If you gargle, it stimulates the vocal cords in the back, just like with humming as well. Whenever you gargle, you also will notice there is a tingling sensation in your mouth too. That tingling is a sign you're stimulating the vagus nerve, and it should be a sign you're doing the right thing.

Gargling doesn't have to be some pretty, exact sequence either. Sometimes gargling very loudly will help with this too, since it helps to push and bring effort forward, which will help stimulate it even more.

One great way to stimulate your vagus nerve with gargling is via filtered water. Saltwater does this too, similar to how it can help with sore throats. Some also might do this in the shower, since it doesn't require you to spend extra time at the sink. If you're a stickler for filtered water, this might not work, but if you know the water in your shower is clean, it shouldn't be a problem.

You have to gargle loudly, and it sounds strange. But, that's the point of it. If you end up laughing, that's even better, since it'll help with stimulating the vagus nerve.

Some people will do this when they need to rinse their mouths out with water, in order to form a habit. The big thing with this is that doing it once won't fix this, but rather you must do this again and again to get the effects of it.

This is one of the best ways to stimulate this neve, but all of the tips listed in here are helpful. We'll also talk about actual exercises you can do to stimulate your vagus nerve naturally, but that'll be in another chapter. For now, consider how you can incorporate these into your lifestyle, and from there you simply do it. It's that simple, and that effective. Consider it, and see the difference it makes within you right away.

Chapter 9:
Vagus Nerve Stimulation, The Medical Process and When You Need It

One part of improving vagal tone is, of course, vagus nerve stimulation. However, this is something you shouldn't look into unless you know for sure you're unable to stimulate your vagus nerve otherwise. It's the only invasive procedure we've discussed so far, and you usually can't get vagus nerve stimulation, or VNS, without medical clearance from a professional.

But, if you know that you've tried all of these and you *still* have an unstimulated vagus nerve, here is the process of vagus nerve stimulation, what it entails, and the risk associated with this as well.

So, what Is It?

Vagus nerve stimulation is a treatment that directly taps not the vagus nerve via electrical impulse generation. So, it's similar to a pacemaker in a sense, except instead of putting it near the heart, it's put near your vagus nerve.

While it doesn't require brain surgery or anything, it does involve you being put under for the procedure to work. Other homeopathic treatments we've discussed don't require this. You don't need anesthesia for gargling or laughing, for example.

However, if your vagus nerve isn't stimulated period, you're going to need this.

The procedure implements a device that sends out pulses that are electrical. Remember, the nervous system communicates with electrical impulses. They will directly signal our vagus nerve in order to stimulate it if it's not working period. If your vagus nerve is overworking though, it'll control it. This can help with your motor functions, your vocal cords, and also sensory functions, and can help with resetting your digestive system so it's properly stimulated.

Basically, all those issues we discussed in the previous chapters that are caused by your vagus nerve can be controlled by this little device. And, in case if you're wondering, it's so small and insignificant you probably won't even notice it's there. This type of treatment isn't for everyone either.

In order to get this kind of treatment, you have to prove that you can't use homeopathic treatments. If you're resistant to those types of treatments, it might not work for you either.

To find out if you qualify for this at all, talk to your doctor. You should remember that this quite invasive, and a more natural approach is usually better for everyone.

Considerations for This Treatment

This procedure is used when you don't have a vagus nerve that's stimulated naturally. So, if you've tried natural methods, but you can't seem to get any results, then this might be for you.

In order to qualify for this kind of procedure, you need to try other forms of treatment before this is even a suggestion.

Some people might also get this if they're resistant to drugs, especially for those with depression that's resistant to that form of treatment. If you've got epilepsy that can't be controlled naturally, this is also an option too.

There are also certain criteria that will make you both available and unavailable for this kind of treatment. If you have only one vagus nerve, for example, you won't be able to get this kind of treatment. If you're already getting stimulation from other procedures, then you can't have this treatment either. If you have heart issues, where you're already using a pacemaker for them, then you can't get this kind of treatment.

Those with arrhythmia also can't get this either, since the heart rate isn't even, and it can ultimately affect the way this plays out.

Some people who have dysautonomia, which means irregular nervous system treatment might not be eligible for this either since it can put too much stress on the entire body.

There are other considerations that people take into account too. If your autonomic nervous system isn't working correctly, you're not eligible either. Some people might also not able to use this if they suffer from asthma or even shortness of breath. If you have ulcers, whether gastric or duodenal ulcers, you might not be qualified for this kind of procedure either.

If you suffer from vasovagal syncope, which is that word which means fainting due to overstimulation of your vagus nerve, you're not qualified for this ether. The obvious reason for that being, it will stimulate your vagus nerve, but if you're sensitive to stimulation of the vagus nerve, it could prove to be a problem for you too.

The best way to figure out whether or not you qualify for this procedure is, of course, to see your doctor regarding it.

What's the Procedure?

If you're qualified for the procedure, then great! If you're wondering what it entails, read on below.

The procedure is very specific, but it's also a quick procedure too. Generally, this takes less than a couple of hours. To do this, you're given general anesthetic, and for the most part, it's similar to outpatient methods for most people. You don't need to stay in the hospital overnight unless there are complications.

Usually, the doctor gives you some medications to take before, or even after surgery. Make sure to take them, since there is a risk for infection and inflammation. But the risk is also quite small compared to other types of procedures that are similar to this. And of course, it's much simpler than mere brain surgery.

The process involves the following: two incisions are made on your left side of the chest, near the upper area, and it's the skin closer to the neck than anything else. The device is placed then right near the area since it's right by the vagus nerve.

At that point, another incision is made near the neck, where you have the skin creases, and from there, you have wires implemented in there. From there, wires will connect towards the pulse generator that's on the chest. These are all put together, and once everything is patched up, then you're good to go! It's that simple, and very effective as well.

How it Stimulates

How does this device stimulate then? It's actually very simple. You have the wires, and the device, and on the device is a very small piece that's incredibly small, and only a few millimeters thick, and a couple of inches long. Some models are even smaller than this, so it's really not even detectable unless you're going through airport security or something that can detect this type of item.

You have a battery added to this, and it can last about 15 years in many cases. It doesn't feel like it's there most of the time, but if you need to replace it, you can.

When the battery runs low, it'll make a sound that means it needs to be replaced. This battery is only located in one of the incisions though.

The stimulator is activated a couple of weeks after it's put in, so it won't be working right away. But, some people might have it activated as soon as it's implanted in the body. It just depends on the circumstance.

As for how much stimulation is there, at first it starts out very low. That's because if your body is sensitive to the stimulation, it might be too much. But over time it might increase, and help to get the vagus nerve to stimulate without its interference. That does happen in some cases.

Over time, the device will configure and increase the output. It's always running, but every once in a while, it'll shut off, so it doesn't waste battery life. After a bit, or with the proper stimulation, it'll turn itself back on.

Patients can stimulate this device themselves if they feel like they need extra stimulation. What they do, is they take that magnetic bracelet that's on their arm, and wave it right over the chest, where the device is implanted, in order to provide more stimulation. The patient is then in complete control of how they'd like to stimulate this device, which means that they control just how much they need to get the proper stimulation necessary.

That's all it is, and it's so simple, but also very effective.

The Pros

There are many benefits to this procedure. If you can't control your vagus nerve by normal means, this is one of the best treatments for this. That's because, with just the wave of your bracelet, you'll have stimulation you might not otherwise get.

It also easily stimulates the vagus nerve. This device is incredibly responsible, meaning that you don't have to worry about it potentially not working or anything, so that's a nice little added touch to it as well.

The procedure is also one of the least invasive in terms of treatments regarding both vagal tones, and also involving stimulating the nervous system. There are other types of treatments you can get that are much more invasive, and it can put you at risk as well. So, this is healthier for you, and better too.

It usually doesn't take all that long to implement either. So, if you're struggling with inflammation, or would like to curb autoimmune diseases, this can readily do it so you're not at the mercy of them.

There are a few downsides you should consider though, since not every surgery has an easy procedure to it.

The Risks and Downsides

The problem with this procedure is that it requires you to have certain criteria. Most of the time, if you're having issues with vagus nerve stimulation and can prove it, you'll get it, but if you're suffering from other health conditions, you might be denied, especially compared to other procedures.

However, there are complications that happen, and initially, you might feel pain when this inserted. That's because it's taking time to adjust. Over time, the pain might dissipate, but many times, if you feel it too much, you might need to get it removed.

Sometimes, this device can have other complications, such as random tiredness, struggling with breathing, issues with swallowing, or other problems. Sometimes, this might be acute, but if it keeps up for very long periods of time, do see your doctor.

Another downside is that MRIs are affected by this device, so if you get those on the regular, please be careful with them.

Most people won't get this type of procedure however since they may respond to drugs and other treatments first. Some people might do better with ECT too rather than this, but again, you should talk to your doctor.

Who can benefit from this?

Well, the obvious is people who suffer from a lack of vagus nerve stimulation, which may result in autoimmune disorder sand breathing issues. But, those with epilepsy that are responsive to the drugs and treatment that you get might actually benefit from this procedure.

Those who have treatment-resistant depression also can befit from this. If you don't want to get ECT, this is a good one, since you can control the device. The procedure does use electricity, and it will improve the symptoms, sometimes gradually. It also has much more success than normal ECT would, so it might be good.

Those who have schizophrenia of any kind, bipolar, delusions, or other degenerative mental health conditions that are severe and can't be alleviated with normal drugs, this is for you.

This is a god procedure for treating the vagus nerve, but do keep in mind this procedure isn't normally covered by insurance if it's treating vagus nerve conditions or depression. But, if it is treating epilepsy, then this might be the perfect treatment for you and might be worth checking out.

Vagus nerve stimulation is a bit of a bigger issue than you might think, and for those who look towards vagus nerve stimulation to treat their conditions, they need to understand that this process does pose serious risks, but it also has many marked health benefits, especially if you're someone who normally doesn't respond to different treatments effectively. It's something to consider, and something which can ultimately benefit you if you would like to try it.

Chapter 10:
Meditation for Stimulating the Vagus Nerve

Did you know that the vagus nerve and meditation are interconnected? That's right, these to activities are intimately connected, and by using meditation, it can help with this.

Meditation is a great practice, mostly because people are stressed out. When we're stressed, it affects our vagus nerve, which of course means that we're constantly stressed, aren't able to breathe properly, can't digest food correctly, and so on.

Meditation lets you sit down and realize what's going on with yourself, sometimes becoming mindful of all you're going through, letting you effectively measure the stress levels there.

Meditation helps you get your attention off of what's going on around you, and instead, brings you into the moment, and makes you face what's happening in the body as well.

How are these connected? What's a good meditation for vagus nerve stimulation? Read on to find out.

The Power of Meditation

Meditation is powerful, no matter how you do it. It's great for vagus nerve stimulation.

In particular, mindfulness meditation is one of the best practices for vagus nerve stimulation.

Mindfulness means that you're becoming aware and know what's going on in the world around you. Sometimes, when we're stressed, our attention is transfixed into that moment, instead of looking at the world around us. But, when we practice meditation, our attention is pulled out from these distracting thoughts, bringing us into the present moment, and feeling better.

Meditation is inexpensive, and in many cases it's free, and it isn't invasive like surgeries or procedures. You can do this wherever you want, whether it be sitting down or walking about, and you can focus on the different aspects of your life.

Meditation is really helpful since it will naturally calm down the body. In particular, loving-kindness and mindfulness meditation are great for improving your vagal tone. Some people also may notice a benefit when they use breathing meditation.

Meditation is a way for you to contemplate whether or not you have problems going on in life too, and also lets you focus on them as well. That way, you're not so obsessed with the problems at hand, and instead, you can have a better focus on the future.

What Meditation Should I Do?

That really ultimately depends on what you're comfortable with. We'll go over each of the types of meditation below, why they're good for you, and whether you should do them or not.

Chanting Meditation

First, you have chanting, chanting, is usually done by using the sound of your mouth, making a vocalization of whatever noise you'd like to make.

This one has the extra benefit of directly stimulating the vagus nerve. One way I like to do this is to sit down, close my eyes, and focus on the sound of my voice. Only focus on that, and when intrusive thoughts and stresses come about, I get rid of them. This is one of the best ways to make sure you're not getting distracted, but also helps with keeping you in check.

Not only that, when you make those sounds, they directly stimulate the vagus nerve. So, you're making it easier to directly stimulate and target it, and you'll feel the difference much more readily.

Breathing Meditation

We'll talk about diaphragmic breathing in the next chapter, but breathing meditation is another form of meditation that has many wonderful benefits. For starters, it's very easy. It requires literally no extra items or money. Just your body, and your breathing.

Not only that, breathing meditation is also incredibly simple to do. To do this, you sit down, close your eyes, and focus on your breathing. You want to take deep breaths in and out, but while you do this, you focus on your breathing, and naturally, relatedly, focus on this.

Don't do anything else but focus on breathing in, and out. Continue to do this and as you notice these intrusive thoughts coming in and rearing their ugly head, you simply acknowledge them and move on.

This form of meditation is a little bit harder for some, since the goal is to focus on your breathing, and if you feel like you're not really able to handle this, start with chant meditation first before you move to this next one, since it can make this much easier, and more powerful.

Mindfulness Meditation

This can tie into the last two, but also is its own separate thing. Mindfulness is a pretty word which means awareness of the situations that are happening at hand, but also not getting hung up on them. It also means acknowledging what the body is doing, rather than getting all into the different intricacies of the body itself.

Mindfulness meditation is something that you should do whenever you're able to. It's so easy, and the beauty of this one is that you can do it anywhere. Some people get a lot out of just the lotus-style meditative breathing, whilst others get a lot out of doing this while they brush their teeth, or take a shower. The idea behind this is pretty simple.

What you need to do, is focus on what you're doing. You'll start to realize that you don't really do this, and that's a fault of all of us as humans. We don't actually sit around and focus on what we're doing, but instead, we go into autopilot the moment we do it.

Autopilot works well for something, but n

However, mindfulness meditation takes
and out of your head, and helps you with f
and the world around you. This can help a
feel like you're not really experiencing
through, and instead, going through the motions.

Many of us do things robotically without even knowing it. Mindfulness meditation is kind of a good kick in the pants, a great way to wake up and smell the roses, and a wonderful way to build an understanding of yourself. This helps stimulate the vagus nerve too because it will help you naturally calm down, help you know exactly what it is that you're doing, and help you become more appreciative of life.

Mindfulness meditation is the easiest of all of these and the most worthwhile of them all. Consider adding this to your repertoire of actions to naturally stimulate your vagus nerve, and see the difference in this right away.

Deep breathing with this is also used too. Some people utilize attentive breathing techniques, which means they're paying attention to how they breathe in order to bring forth calmness and understanding of the different aspects of their body.

Sometimes, mindfulness is the perfect way to naturally relieve stress. What many of us don't realize, is that we're incredibly stressed, that our lives are too full of hustle and bustle to do much about it. But, by breathing in deeply, becoming mindful of what's happening around you, and practicing meditation, you'll be happier too.

...ype of meditation that'll help you, is, of course, loving-...dness meditation. This is a type of meditation that forces us to focus on the love, adoration, and care we provide to others.

You can combine this with yoga, or do it on your own. For starters, take a moment and think about the love you give to others. Think about the energies you put forth to one person. Now, imagine that same person giving you that same energy.

From there think about the love you can give to the next person. Figure out the love you can give to two people, and from there, as you inhale, push your hands out, and focus on the love that you have within you with your hands. When you exhale out, close your eyes and imagine your love going outwards. You can move your hands along with this for better imagery.

You can then think about someone who is going through something similar to you. Think about friends who are stressed out, who aren't sure of what to do, and imagine giving them the love, compassion and understanding within you. This is a great way to feel these same feelings.

From there, you should think about how you can feel this same sense of compassion and understanding for yourself, and how you can practice this.

This type of meditation is something that you can use which spans all throughout the world. You can from there extend towards a bigger realm of understanding, and that, in turn, is incredibly therapeutic.

This type of meditation is amazing for your vagus nerve. Most people don't even realize how they don't show enough love, and how they can improve on their own stress by engaging in meditation.

How to Use Meditation to Stimulate Your Vagus Nerve

How do you use it?

Well, I personally like to, when I'm stressed out after a long day of work or after something that's stressful, sit down somewhere, take a deep breath, and from there focus on what stimulates the mind, and focus on yourself.

From there, you should focus on three things that calm you down. Focus on one of these at a time. Become mindful of all the different aspects of life happening around you. For example, if you're in the office, you should focus on the sounds heard, the visuals seen, or even the various scents that are around you. Be mindful of your body placement, and how it sits too.

From there, breathe in, and breathe out. I suggest using deep breathing since it helps with focusing on the energy of the body.

If you notice yourself feeling relaxed, then awesome! Keep on going, and from there if you really feel good, from there go back to whatever you're doing, and be mindful of how you're feeling. Be mindful of what you just did, and don't just ignore those feelings.

Every time you're stressed out, you should be down, close your eyes, and for a few minutes just be there, and of course be mindful. This type of meditation will help with stimulating the vagus nerve, ensuring things will get better, and to help with improving your health and wellness over time.

There is a lot of benefit you can get with this, and a lot of use for this. If you're curious about what meditation can do for stimulating the vagus nerve, I suggest trying it, since it's a simple, yet effective means to help with making you feel more comfortable not only with yourself, but also with different aspects.

Sometimes it's scary being honest with the way that you feel, and the mindfulness you're experiencing. But, it's important to understand that this does happen and that you'll be happier just being honest with yourself, and you'll be amazed at the difference this makes, and the stimulation this provides to your vagus nerve too.

Chapter 11:
Breathing, and How it helps Your Vagus Nerve

One way to naturally stimulate the vagus nerve is via breathing. Did you know the right kind of breathing helps immensely with stimulating the vagus nerve? How does that work though? Well, you'll find out here. Breathing, combined with meditation, or even on its own, is one of the best ways to stimulate your vagus nerve, and we'll tap into why that is, and how it helps in this chapter.

Why Breathing?

First, I want you to do an exercise. Sit down, close your eyes, and take a nice, deep breath in through the nose, noticing the belly expanding rather than the chest. From there, breathe out, and notice how the belly contracts.

Did you notice as you dd this how your body slowly relaxed, how your heart rate settled, and maybe you feel a little less anxious?

Well, that's an example of diaphragmic breathing, and how it stimulates the body.

Diaphragmic breathing, or deep breathing, is breathing with your diaphragm as the focus, rather than the chest. When you breathe from your chest, you're not supplying the body with oxygen-rich air, and many times, it will deprive the body of this. Breathing from your chest is how hyperventilation happens, and in some cases, brings about anxiety in some people.

When you breathe from your diaphragm, you'll feel it, and your body will naturally relax. That's because you're activating the parasympathetic nervous system. Most people discount this form of breathing as a means to relieve stress, but it's very important not just for stress relief, but stimulating your vagus nerve.

When you do this though, you must understand that not all forms of breathing are equal. You have to breathe in through the nose, and from there, feel your belly expand. Sometimes, I like to hold my hand there in order to help facilitate the feeling of this. From there, I will notice how the stomach grows, and then flattens with this.

When you do this, you should notice your heart rate, breathing rate, and your body's general wellness change. Some people report a change in heartrate when that happens. Others will report a change in the way their breathing occurs. Some people will also notice their bodies general relax over time. This is a type of breathing that can help you with improving vagal tone, since it's naturally touching on this, and it will help with stimulating your parasympathetic nervous system.

When you breathe quickly, that'll stimulate your sympathetic nervous system. That's important for physical activities, but if you're always breathing that quickly, you'll force yourself into a panic attack. It gives the body the sign it has to be ready for action, whereas when you breathe in deeply, it'll naturally stimulate your vagus nerve, so it'll help with making sure your body is taken care of, and the vagus nerve is properly touched upon.

Deep breathing is essential to general health, wellness, and happiness.

Does Deep Breathing Help in Other Ways?

Of course! Deep breathing isn't just for vagus nerve stimulation. It helps with a lot of the various aspects of your body, and we'll talk a little bit here about how deep breathing helps you.

When you breathe in deeply, you'll provide more oxygen to the body. Oxygen is important, because it helps recover from hard exercises, and it also helps the body feel less stressed over time.

It reduces the exertion that's in the body, and it allows for you to get better sleep, and help stimulate creativity, and provide mental clarity as well. If you have brain fog happening, breathing deeply can help with this.

It also naturally relaxes the body. So, after a day filled with stress, it's the perfect means to help chill out after a very long day.

But, along with that is overall health. When you breathe in deeply, you're supplying oxygen to the body. That means, all physical activities within the body are better. It'll help with digestion, secretion, nervous system function, and also help with your heartrate.

It'll reduce the instances of vasovagal syncope, and also help with reducing inflammation in the body. It can boost immunity too, and red blood cell function.

Simply put, just by breathing in deeper, it'll help with improving your body's overall health. You'll start to feel the difference right away, and improve on these aspects too.

However, when you do deep breathing, you need to make sure that you're breathing with the whole body, and not just with your mouth. When you breathe from your mouth, you'll notice you'll feel less anxious. When you breathe from your diaphragm, you'll stay more grounded, and you might even notice your diaphragm moving, and if you take your blood pressure, you'll notice it'll lower too.

In the body, diaphragmic breathing does other things too. When you breathe from the diaphragm, it triggers acetylcholine release, which helps with reducing stress in the body. It also reduces cortisol rates. Cortisol is the stress chemical, so in general, it'll promote the parasympathetic activity, and relaxation.

It also will take the inflammation system, so those with autoimmune disorders will notice the difference right away. It can reduce further inflammation, and also help with inflammation in the future too.

Your body will feel inner calmness. When you breathe from your diaphragm, it is controlled breathing. This gives you a sense of control over yourself, your emotions, and the adaptations that you have psychologically, and it'll allow you to express yourself better, and you'll notice you'll feel a lot calmer in even the worst of situations.

You'll also notice a better sense of well-being after you breathe from your diaphragm. It helps you in general and makes you feel great. It helps on many fronts and will benefit you greatly.

Using Diaphragmic Breathing with Meditation

Now, remember in the previous chapter when we said using diaphragmic breathing with meditation is possible? We'll discuss that there.

The best way to do it is either through breathing meditation where you sit down and focus on your breathing, or even, after a long day with many meetings, close your eyes, and from there, breathe in deeply for five seconds, and then breathe out for 10 seconds. Once you start breathing in, you might notice the heartrate increasing, and as you breathe out, from there it'll decrease. This helps to naturally stabilize the body, and increase both intention and attention.

Doing this on its own, or even just with your body in different places, such as in the shower, or even when walking around can prove to be incredibly beneficial.

I like to do this sometimes in the shower. I'll close my eyes, and become mindful of the body as I breathe in deeply, and from there, breathe out as well. I become mindful of the world around me, and my breathing, which in turn will change the way I handle various aspects of life. Diaphragmic breathing helps with handling all of the different changes, and aspects of life.

One great way to utilize this type of breathing is with a guided meditation. Sometimes, turning on a guided meditation before you begin will help you focus. I've done this before, and it helps immensely with keeping me grounded and focused. It also promotes the right mindset when doing this.

Sometimes, guided meditations also include breathing too, and you can do diaphragmic breathing while following along with this.

Sometimes, when you've got a few moments of downtime, diaphragmic breathing can be used. I like to do it sometimes when I'm in the car on the way home from work and I'm stuck in traffic. Just make sure you're paying attention to the road as you do it.

I also think using diaphragmic breathing with other meditations is incredibly beneficial. For example, I like to do this with loving-kindness meditation. That's because, as I'm experiencing the love flowing in, I can breathe in deeply, and from there as I send my love out to others, I can from there breathe out in a deep, and controlled manner.

No matter how you do this, no matter what type of breathing you do, breathing from your diaphragm will change things. Instead of breathing from your chest, breathe with a deeper focus on the way your diaphragm moves, and how it goes up and then goes down.

You'll feel the difference right away. You can do this during downtime as well. If you have a few minutes to relax, you can do this, and it can markedly help too.

For Those Who are Busy a Lot

I get it, a lot of us may not have much downtime to do this. But that's where breaks come in. during your breaks at work, you can use diaphragmic breathing in order to ground yourself. If you don't have the time or the drive to do meditations, you can use this. To do it, you can sit down in your chair, close your eyes, and from there, just breathe from your diaphragm for about 5-10 minutes at a time. Sometimes, having some music that plays in the background helps too with calming down, especially if you live a life where you're constantly moving from one point to another.

I also think after that, take a moment to not do something super mentally stimulating, such as listen to a song. This way, you're turning off the sympathetic nervous system for a moment or so, and from there, letting the parasympathetic nervous system, and the vagus nerve, work together in order to help relax and stimulate the body in a relaxed manner.

Sometimes, after a long meeting doing this will help ground you. It's also great to do after a long day of work, before your drive home. Even just doing this right before you go to bed is a wonderful way to help stimulate your vagus nerve, promote sleep, and reduce inflammation.

If you have trouble implementing this, try to incorporate a schedule into this. Schedules are a great way to improve your wellness and happiness's and to stimulate the vagus nerve. I know a lot of people struggle with schedules, but they can prove to be quite wonderful, and are helpful for even the busiest people. Scheduling out just five minutes of diaphragmic breathing is wonderful, helpful for people, and can improve your mental state too. You don't have to sit around and do an hour of meditation. Though, it might help you in some cases.

When looking to stimulate your vagus nerve in simple ways, this is one of the best ways to do it. It'll clear the mind, and if you combine with meditation, you'll see the difference right away. Most don't realize the power this has, but as you work with this, you'll feel the difference right away, and from there stimulate your vagus nerve properly, and better than ever before. If nothing else, it'll help with meditation, and make it possible for you to open up the neural pathways, and activate your parasympathetic nervous system.

Chapter 12:
Practical Exercises to Stimulate the Vagus Nerve

Finally, let's talk practical exercises that'll change your vagus nerve's state. Exercising is very important for the body, but did you know it could stimulate the vagus nerve too/ here, we'll discuss practical exercises that'll stimulate your vagus nerve, and some of the different aspects that go along with this type of nerve.

Yoga

First, let's talk about yoga. Yoga is one of the simplest exercises to stimulate the vagus nerve, but not only that, it's wonderful for promoting bodily relaxation and general wellness.

Yoga requires you to do small positions, whether it be downward dog, different hand and foot positions, or even a simple lotus position. What you do while doing this, is focus on your breathing. You're encouraged to have even, soft breathing from your diaphragm, and also to hold the position, feeling your muscles at first tense, but then relax as you hold it for longer.

Yoga is one of the single best ways to stimulate your vagus nerve. It's simple, it doesn't take much, to begin with it, and you don't have to do it for a long period of time. It is a form of exercise, and it's calming.

But, don't underestimate yoga. It can be quite powerful. Some people struggle with it, simply because it's oftentimes long, and you might not be used to these various positions. It's quite freeing though, and it liberates you.

If you're someone who only has a little bit of time for physical activity every day, then try yoga. There are many variants to it too, many positions that'll stimulate your vagus nerve just by doing them and holding them, and that's something that most don't realize.

The Power of Yoga Nidra

One aspect of yoga that's worth mentioning is yoga Nidra. This is one of the best types of yoga practices since it lets you naturally restore your body, along with your mind via unlocking and touching upon your parasympathetic nervous system. It is a slow practice, but incredibly powerful, and very helpful for building better wellness, and understanding of your vagus nerve.

How do you do it through? Well first, you want to get int a comfortable position, whether with a blanket or a mat. From there close your eyes, and start to breathe. Start to become aware of your breathing, and space and the feelings you possess. From there, sit there, and hold that position, focusing on the breathing.

You can lay down, you can have your legs crossed, you can have them sit up. Literally, just sit down, and from there, relax. This is nourishing, this is filling, and it's a relaxing experience too.

Hold the position for as long as you want, but usually, about 30 minutes is more than enough.

The Power of Stretching

Let's talk about stretching. This doe tie into yoga, but if you combine diaphragmic breathing with yoga. Doing this as you do a mall stretch, it'll benefit you in a ton of different ways. For starters, most people don't stretch nearly enough, and it shows. Most people aren't flexible, and it affects how they end up faring in life. Many get injured due to a lack of stretching.

But, it's more than that. Stretching is powerful. Stretching is used in order to help naturally stimulate the body, and make movement simple. There is a lot you can get from this, and a lot you can get out of this. Most people don't realize that when they stretch, they're not only releasing tensions within the muscles, but they're also focusing their breathing so it's simple, and yet very effective.

A lot of people don't stretch enough, so that tension sits there. But, a way to naturally start up the parasympathetic nervous system and activate et vagus nerve is to do just this. Sitting down, stretching out your body, and working on this helps promote relaxation and wellness, and from there will stimulate your entire body in its own way.

Plus, it feels amazing too. Most people don't stretch enough, and they'll realize as they do this, that they really need to. Sometimes having calming music, and focusing on your breathing changes this.

You also don't have to hold the stretches for very long. About 10-12 seconds suffices.

Try touching your toes, stretching your arms behind your head, pushing them up and holding your arms in the air, or even just moving towards your foot will help with this. There is a lot of benefits to be had with stretching, and a lot of wonderful things to do with this. You'll be shocked, you'll be amazed, and most of all, you'll be quite happy with the power of this small exercise, and you'll feel invigorated for whatever is to come next for you in the future.

Consider stretching right before you begin your day, or at the end of the night, and see how it helps you feel during the day, and you'll feel your vagus nerve stimulate almost immediately.

Weight Training

Weight training might seem weird to do in order to stimulate the vagus nerve, but it does work. That's because, when you lift weights, it is changing the speed of the body. Plus, through the power of repetition, you get your body to relax. A lot of people think lifting weights is only for big, burly people, but that isn't the case.

Ever just doing a few sets of curls will change the way your body feels, and your vagus nerve. So many people also think they need to start off with a heavy weight right away, but that isn't the case. I suggest just progressively overloading over time if you want to see physical gains, but you must understand that weight training is a relaxing process, and you must breathe as you do it. You need to breathe in deeply in order to help with pushing the oxygen around to help you with strenuous exercise. So yes, pick up that dumbbell, and try it. You'll feel the difference right away.

HIIT Workouts

HIIT, or "high intensity interval training" is a form of workouts that require you to do a lot in a very small period of time. Sometimes, this involves sprinting, other times this can be pushups, sit-ups, or other exercises. The main goal behind this is to do a lot in a little bit of time, and through spurts.

These sprits are what cause vagus nerve stimulation. The vagus nerve is usually not stimulated if you're constantly stressed out, but the periods of stress, and then relaxation will kick the vagus nerve into gear, helping it activate whenever it's needed.

HIIT workouts are also great because they are oftentimes very easy to do. No matter what it is that you do, you'll feel the difference in these immediately.

A lot of people don't realize that HIIT is also very short in terms of workouts. Some people can get these done within a half hour or so, and that's their workout for the day. But HIIT is great because it lets you get a great workout, but also lets you improve your own personal wellness, and health too.

It's a great way to get in shape, so it's something you should consider if you're looking to improve your physical fitness.

Walking

Walking is a great option if you're not into going to the gym to lift, or you don't want to spend time doing HIIT or yoga. Walking is a good habit to get into because it stimulates your body and helps with physical fitness and wellness. Your vagus nerve will get stimulated with walking, especially if you live a sedentary lifestyle.

I think walking for 30 minutes a day is ideal, especially if you're unable to do this otherwise. Sometimes, walking while on your breaks is a great way to do this, and walking also lets you improve on your own personal health and wellness. You want to do this to help with your physical fitness, and walking is a good start, especially if you're not active otherwise.

Jogging is also another good one because this can help with deep breathing. A lot of people, when they start, will get into the habit of breathing with short breaths, but that won't work here. This can actually make it hard to run, and you might pass out. With jogging, you want to make sure that you're breathing in a slow, deep, and even manner, and focus on this. This will help with your vagus nerve, and also help you get into the habit of breathing deeply. You can also do running with this, but it's more high-intensity and might be harder to engage in deep breathing otherwise.

Jumping

Again, another form of cardio that's great, but, your vagus nerve will love it. Jumping jacks, burpees, and other jumping exercises are good because it will help with improving circulation, which can help with blood pressure and your vagal tone.

When you jump too, be mindful of your breathing. Try to do it with deep breathing, and you'll notice it's a much harder workout, but you'll feel the difference. It also increases blood flow, blood pressure, and heart rate as well.

Your vagus nerve will thank you for this, and you'll be able to, with jumping too, improve on your own personal health and wellness too.

Aerobics

Aerobics is another higher-intensity exercise, but there are variants that aren't as extensive or intensive as others. Zumba tends to be on the more intensive side, but there are different classes you can try. However, there are even different kinds of aerobics exercises you can do, such as water aerobics, weight training, cycling, and even yoga.

All of these when combined, are wonderful for vagus nerve stimulation and are great for the body. You'll be amazed and surprised at how helpful this can be for the body, and how you can use these to help improve your vagus nerve. They encourage you to breathe during these too, which encourages deep breathing, and thereby vagus nerve stimulation.

Swim it Out!

Swimming is a great aerobic exercise too, and if you're not a fan of jogging or running, or weight training, swimming is good.

That's because it actually helps in many different ways. For starters, you're submerging your head, which stimulates the mammalian diving reflex, which includes your vagus nerve. It also pushes you to control your breathing as you move. You need to hold your breath, but also move through the water, and it's a combination of both of those things which provides you with the correct vagus nerve stimulation.

It also will help improve your bodily movement. That's because, you're moving about, and this encourages blood flow too. You'll notice that as you begin with this, at first, it's hard to do, but over time, you'll get better with this. It's a wonderful form of cardio, and it's wonderful for properly stimulating the vagus nerve.

Dancing

Finally, we have dancing. Dancing is a great form of self-expression for starters, and even if you're being silly, it can help you feel much better about yourself. Dance is wonderful because it helps you improve your physical fitness, get the blood flow moving, and help you stay active and fun.

There are so many different kinds of dance classes these days too. You can do Zumba or other forms of dancing. Some people even like ballet dancing because it requires control, and this can stimulate the vagus nerve. They're fun to do, and they encourage you to move, control your breathing, and also let you express yourself.

Even silly interpretive dancing helps. After all, if it can make you laugh, that naturally stimulates the vagus nerve, and that's a wonderful, fun way to do this. Dancing is great, and it lets you feel good about yourself. Definitely consider dancing next time you want to properly express yourself and feel good.

When it comes to stimulating the vagus nerve, these are all practice activities to help with stimulating the vagus nerve. Your vagus nerve is very important because it lets you relax the body and helps curb inflammation. But, while these exercises are great for stimulating this, it also helps with getting the body moving, which increases vagal tone. It can also help offset obesity, diabetes, and other conditions related to weight.

Your vagus nerve does benefit from exercise, and here, we discussed why and how it happens, and the benefits of this.

Conclusion

Your vagus nerve is an important part of you, and you should take proper care in order to stimulate this. That's because, if you don't properly do it, it can cause a lot of trouble for you, both now and in the future.

If you already suffer from inflammation, autoimmune conditions, or heart and respiratory issues, you should look at your vagus nerve in order to figure out the culprit behind these. Your vagus nerve is important, and you should make sure you take some time in order to ensure you work towards proper health and wellness from this.

With that being said, look at your body. Do you sometimes feel like you're always stressed out? Do you have autoimmune conditions and inflammatory problems? If the answer is yes, your vagus nerve might be to blame for this. In that case, you need to take the right steps to properly stimulate it, and from there, have a healthier body. Your vagus nerve is important, and don't forget about it either.

Printed in Great Britain
by Amazon

37230748R00068